Navigating the Channels

of Traditional Chinese Medicine

Yitian Ni, O.M.D.

with

Richard L. Rosenbaum

Cover and Interior Graphics
Zemin Zhang

Published in the United States by the Oriental Medicine Center, San Diego.

First Edition
Fourth Printing
Complementary Medicine Press
ISBN 0-9673034-3-5

To the memory of my mother, Binqing Xu

About the Author

Yitian Ni has been teaching and practicing TCM since late 60's , both in the PRC and the U.S.A. She carries on a tradition of medical practice, which has been handed down through many generations of her family. Dr. Ni graduated from and, for many years, taught at the Nanjing College of Traditional Chinese Medicine. Her education includes both Western medicine and TCM, which has allowed her participate in scientific research, publication of several books and numerous papers.

Her teaching career includes positions at the Nanjing College of Traditional Chinese Medicine, the Intentional Training Center of Acupuncture and Herbs (jointly sponsored by the World Health Organization and the Ministry of Health of the PRC), Academy of Traditional Chinese Medicine, Beijing (PRC), visiting professor at the Ministry of Health, Capital Hospital UAE (United Arab Emirates), academic dean and professor of the American Institute of Oriental Medicine and professor of the Pacific College of Oriental Medicine in San Diego, California. She currently teaches and practices in San Diego, California.

Contents

Preface

In the words of Li Yan, a famous doctor of Ming Dynasty, "To practice acupuncture without knowing channels is like working at night without a candle, or sailing without navigation". Traditionally, Channel Theory has been the primary theoretical basis for acupuncture. Without a firm understanding of its dynamics and application, an entire dimension of powerfully effective treatment strategies is unavailable to the practitioner.

Throughout my teaching career, Channel Theory has been one of my great enthusiasms. Over the years, I became a specialist in the instruction of Channel Theory, which I apply extensively in my practice. Today, when I re-read the <u>Huang Di Nei Jing</u>, the Su Wen and Ling Shu's statements on the value of Channel Theory, I appreciate so much more the truth of its assertions.

While teaching in American schools of Oriental Medicine I observed that, in an effort to provide students with sound diagnostic and treatment principles, there is a tendency to emphasize Zang Fu theory. This satisfactorily addresses the needs of the herbalist, but it subordinates those of the acupuncturist.

My students have always found my presentation of Channel Theory fascinating, and enormously helpful in clinical situations. They often ask me for special or "secret" points to treat certain diseases, thinking these will help them get a "short cut." This is a fallacy. Just as it is much more difficult to become a real healer than a technician, an acupuncturist must know more than just the points. While creative ideas and intuition play an important role in developing treatment strategies, there must be a sound theoretical basis on which to draw.

Until now, the texts available to American TCM instructors and students treated Channel Theory in a relatively cursory manner. It was clear to me that a systematic, comprehensive text, which could serve as both teaching tool and practitioner's reference, was missing from the literature.

This book is unique in its approach, as it groups the regular, divergent, tendinomuscular channel, and luo collateral of each channel together for easy comparison. Their pathways are carefully detailed and presented in clear charts in the same location, to allow the reader the ability to grasp the entire concept of each channel's areas of influence. The eight extra channels are treated in the same comprehensive manner.

All the information is organized in an easy-to-use manner, which gives the book the flexibility to function as either an academic text or a clinical reference. Each channel has its own chapter, containing key points for reference, pathways, associated organs, intersecting points, TCM physiology and pathology, including the regular, divergent, tendinomuscular channels, and the luo collaterals. The clinical application include classical and modern point combinations and commentary.

The patients in all case studies are from my private practice, and represent both common ailments and many intractable disorders American acupuncturists are likely to encounter. These cases have been carefully selected to demonstrate not only the application of channel theory but to give insight into the complexities and dynamics which are encountered in clinical situations. This presentation allows the reader to follow the diagnostic thought processes which brings Channel Theory to life, and generate potent treatment strategies.

It is my belief that the material presented has something to offer TCM practitioners of every level. For the student it provides a firm foundation and systematic approach to Channel Theory, for the young practitioner it will serve for theoretical review and as a clinical tool, and the for the established doctor of Oriental medicine, it is hoped that the advanced theoretical applications and case studies will serve as a stimulus to refining their skills and improving patient care.

August 1996
San Diego, California

Dr. Yitian Ni, O.M.D., L.Ac.

Acknowledgments

The author wishes to express gratitude to the following people: to Don Goddard and Dinesh Quatrochi for their valuable assistance in editing and proof reading; to Zemin Zhang for preparation of the graphics and cover.

The Theory of Channels and Collaterals

Qi and Blood are circulated to the entire body through a specific system, which is comprised of the channels and collaterals. Qi is defined as the refined substance which, as it circulates through the body, manifests and maintains the body's normal functions. Blood is the vital nutrient substance which nourishes the body.

The channel system is divided into two parts: channels and collaterals. In describing the movement and activities of Qi and Blood in the body, the flow of water is often used as a metaphor. The channels are likened to seas, large rivers, and lakes. They are the primary portion of the system. The collaterals are described as smaller rivers and streams, or as branches of the channels. Together they form a network that internally connects the organs, and externally connects the muscles, joints, tissues, and skin.

I. The Functions of the Channels and Collaterals

The theory of channels and collaterals is the guiding principle of acupuncture practice. Together with the theories of the Zang/Fu, Qi, Blood, Body Fluid, and the Four Diagnostic Methods, they constitute the fundamental theory of Traditional Chinese Medicine. The general functions of the channels and collaterals can be summarized as follows:

1. *Integrate the whole body*. The channels and collaterals provide a network which a) connects the Zang and Fu organs one to another, b) connects the interior to the exterior, and c) links each part of the body to every other part, creating an organic whole.

2. *Circulate the Qi and Blood*. The channels and collaterals provide a passage for the circulation of the Qi and Blood, so that a) the organs and tissues can be nourished and lubricated, b) their functions can be regulated, and c) a relative equilibrium of normal life activities can be maintained.

3. *Demonstrate the location of disorders*. The channels and collaterals can provide diagnostic information. When one organ or part of the body is diseased, the pathogenic effect can be transmitted in another area, and meanwhile be reflected on the body surface through the channel system. For example, if the lung is diseased, the pathogens can be transmitted to the large intestine, resulting in a tenderness, or other abnormality on the body surface along the Lung and Large Intestine Channels. The system will also reflect a disorder of one area to another. For example, if a patient feels stomach pain and chest stuffiness, it may be reflected at Pc 6. This may indicate a disorder of the Pericardium Channel. If there is tenderness or swelling at St 36 or LI 11, it may suggest that the patient has indigestion or diarrhea. If there is tenderness at UB 12, it may indicate that pathogenic Wind Cold has invaded the body.

4. *Transmit the needling sensation*. When acupoints are stimulated, the needling sensation can be transported along the channel system to the diseased area. When properly applied, this function regulates and activates the flow of Qi, balances Yin and Yang, and restores the normal function of the organs and channels. For instance, by stimulating Pc 6, stomach pain and vomiting can be stopped.

II. The Components of The Channels and Collaterals

The *Channel System* is comprised of the twelve Regular Channels, twelve Divergent Channels, twelve Tendinomuscular Channels, twelve Cutaneous Regions, and the Eight Extraordinary channels.

The *Collateral System* is comprised of sixteen Major Luo Collaterals, the Grandson Collaterals (minute branches), the Superficial Collaterals, and the Blood Collaterals.

Nomenclature of the Channel System

1. The traditional name of each of the twelve Regular Channels describes three important aspects of the channel: a) the name of the organ to which it pertains, b) the Yin or Yang nature and its pattern of distribution, (i.e., whether it circulates on the medial or lateral, the anterior or posterior aspect of the body), and c) a designation as either a *hand or foot* channel, indicating whether it circulates on either the arm or leg.
2. Each of the Divergent, Tendinomuscular Channels, the Cutaneous Regions, and Major Luo Collaterals shares the name of the Regular Channel of which it is a branch.
3. Each of the Eight Extraordinary Channels has its own name which mainly indicates its function.

Explanation of Tai Yang, Shao Yang, Yang Ming and Tai Yin, Shao Yin, Jue Yin

Channels	Distribution	Quantity of Qi and Blood[1]
Tai Yang	Lateroposterior aspect of the four extremities, posterior aspect of the body and head,	More Blood, less Qi
Shao Yang	Center of the lateral aspect of the four extremities, lateral aspect of the body,	Less Blood, more Qi
Yang Ming	Lateroanterior aspect of the four extremities, front of the face, forehead and trunk	More Qi, more Blood
Tai Yin	Medioanterior aspect of the four extremities, abdomen, chest	More Qi, less Blood
Shao Yin	Medioposterior aspect of the four extremities, abdomen, chest	Less Blood, more Qi
Jue Yin	Center of the medial aspect of the four extremities, abdomen and chest	More Blood, less Qi.

III. The Characteristics of the Channel System

The Twelve Channel System

The Twelve Channel System consists of the Twelve Regular Channels, the Twelve Divergent Channels, the Twelve Tendinomuscular Channels, and the Twelve Cutaneous Regions.

---

[1] This information comes from the *Nei Jing Su Wen* (Plain Questions) chapter 24. It should be noted that in the *Nei Jing, Ling Shu*, (Spiritual Axis) Chapter 65 it states that the Tai Yin has more Blood, less Qi, Shao Yin has more Blood, less Qi, Jue Yin has more Qi, less Blood.

Key points

- The Twelve Regular Channels are the main portion of the system. They play the most important role in the whole of channel theory. There are six pairs of Yin and Yang Channels which form a specific relationship with each other, externally and internally. The Yin Channels are said to "pertain" to the Zang organs, and be "connected" to the Fu organs of their Yang paired channels. The Yang Channels are said to "pertain" to the Fu organs, and be "connected" to the Zang organs of their Yin paired channels. Their distribution and connection follow specific patterns on the body surface.
- The Twelve Divergent Channels are branches of the Regular Channels. They mainly reinforce the connection among the Zang/Fu organs, especially between those organs which are paired through the channel relationships.
- The Twelve Tendinomuscular Channels are external branches of the Regular Channels. Their several functions include reinforcing the connection between the joints, muscles, tendons and ligaments, and maintaining normal articulation. They integrate the body surface.
- The Twelve Cutaneous Regions are the most external portion of the Regular Channels. Their function is to circulate Qi and Blood to the body surface, nourish the skin and pores, and protect the body from being attacked by external pathogens.

A. The Twelve Regular Channels

Characteristics:

1. They are distributed symmetrically (bilaterally) over the entire body. Each has its own regular pathway, which includes an internal and an external course.
2. They are organized into six Yin and Yang pairs, creating an internal/external relationship. Each channel pertains to one organ and is connected to the organ of its paired channel. For instance, the Heart Channel of Hand Shao Yin pertains to the heart and connects with the small intestine. This further demonstrates the internal/external relationship.
3. Their course and distribution accord with the theory of Yin and Yang, as it applies to the areas of the body. The distribution of six Yin Channels is mainly on the medial aspect of the extremities, and the anterior of the trunk. The three Yin Channels of the Hand run from the chest to the hands, while the three Yin Channels of the Foot run from the foot to the chest. The distribution of the Yang Channels is mainly on the lateral aspect of the extremities, the back, and the head and face. The three Yang Channels of the Hand run from the hand to the head and face, while the three Yang Channels of the Foot run from the head and face to the foot.
4. There are several important connections of the Yin and Yang Channels. a) The six Yang Channels meet at the head and face, b) the six Yin Channels meet in the chest, c) all the Yin and Yang Channels of the Hand meet at the hand, d) and all the Yin and Yang Channels of the Foot meet at the foot.
5. The circulation of Qi and Blood through the twelve Regular Channels is endless. According to Chapter 16, "Chapter of Nutritive Qi," of the Nei Jing Ling Shu (Spiritual Axis), the sequence of Nutritive Qi circulation is: Lung → Large Intestine → Stomach → Spleen → Heart → Small Intestine → Urinary Bladder → Kidney → Pericardium → San Jiao → Gall Bladder → Liver, then back to the Lung.
6. Their circulatory functions are to distribute and regulate Qi and Blood, and harmonize and balance the of the organs and the channels themselves.
7. Each of the channels has its own exclusive points where the Qi and Blood converge on the body surface. There are 361 points all together. Each of the points has its own name. A point's name indicates its function, location, or both.
8. Each of the channels has its own pathological symptoms and signs which are important as a guide for acupuncture practice. Channel pathology is also a complement to Zang Fu pathology. The following is excerpted from Chapter 10, "Chapter of Channels," Nei Jing, Ling Shu, (Spiritual Axis):
   The Yin Channels dominate the disorders of their pertaining organs.

a) The Lung Channel dominates the disorders of the Lung.
b) The Heart Channel dominates the disorders of the Heart.
c) The Pericardium Channel dominates the disorders of the Pericardium.
d) The Spleen Channel dominates the disorders of the Spleen.
e) The Liver Channel dominates the disorders of the Liver.
f) The Kidney Channel dominates the disorders of the Kidney.

The Yang Channels dominate the disorders of the body's other structures and fluids:
a) The Large Intestine Channel dominates the disorder of Jin and Ye (body fluids).
b) The Small Intestine Channel dominates the disorders of Ye (body fluids).
c) The San Jiao Channel dominates the disorders of Qi.
d) The Stomach Channel dominates the disorders of blood.
e) The Gall Bladder Channel dominates the disorders of the bone.
f) The Urinary Bladder Channel dominates the disorders of the tendons and ligaments.

Clinical Applications of the Twelve Regular Channels

The clinical applications of the Twelve Regular Channels are based on two principles:
1. The points of each channel will affect its own areas of distribution.
2. All the points, regardless of their channel, can be used for local disorders, e.g., symptoms at the site of the point.

The points of the Twelve channels can be divided into to two categories:
1. *Points on the four extremities, especially those below the knee and elbow.* The points on the four extremities generally have a greater area of influence than those on the trunk, face, and head. This influence can be summarized by the expression *the farther the further.* For example, Stomach Channel points on the foot affect the head and face, those on the legs exert an influence on the abdomen and stomach, while the points on the thigh have only a local effect.
2. *Points on the trunk, face and head.* The influence of these points is usually limited to local disorders. This can be summarized by the expression *the nearer the closer.* For example, UB 1 and St 1 are mainly used for eye disorders, while St 26 and Sp 14 are mainly used for constipation and diarrhea.

The basic principles of clinical application for the Twelve Regular Channels also apply to their branch systems, the Twelve Divergent, Twelve Tendinomuscular, and Twelve Cutaneous Regions.

Summary of the Clinical Applications of the Points on the Four Extremities

Channel	Name	Common Applications for Three Channels	Individual Channel Disorders
3 Yin Channels of the Hand	Lung	Chest Disorders	Lung, throat, nose, Exterior Syndromes.
	Pericardium		Mental, heart, stomach
	Heart		Mental, heart, eye

Channel	Name	Common Applications for Three Channels	Individual Channel Disorders
3 Yang Channels of the Hand	Large Intestine	Face, head, sense organ disorder, febrile diseases	Front of the face and head.
	Small Intestine		Occipital area and nape, scapula region, mental illness.
	San Jiao		Temporal region and sides of the head and face, hypochondriac region.
3 Yang Channels of Foot	Stomach	Mental disorders, febrile diseases, eye disorders	Front of the face and head, digestive system
	Urinary Bladder		Occipital area, nape, back and lumbar region.
	Gall Bladder		Temporal region, side of the head and face, hypochondriac region, hip.
3 Yin Channels of the Foot	Spleen	Urogenital, abdomen and chest disorders	Spleen and stomach
	Kidney		Kidney, lung and throat
	Liver		Liver and Gall Bladder

B. The Twelve Divergent Channels

Characteristics:
1. They share the same name as the Regular Channels of which they are a branch. They supplement the Regular Channels, and emphasizes the circulation of Qi and Blood in the interior of the body. When they circulate in the body cavity, most of the Divergent Channels join with their pertaining organs first, then connect with the organ of their paired channels. In this manner, the bonds between paired Zang and Fu organs and Yin/Yang channels are strengthened and reinforced..
2. They are organized into six Yin and Yang pairs. Each pair circulates together, either on a parallel pathway, or actually joining together. Their distribution is different from the twelve Regular Channels in that they all run from the extremities to the truck, face and head[1].
3. Their distribution can be summarized in four words: *separating* from the Regular Channel, *entering* the body cavity, *emerging* from the body cavity, and *converging* with the Regular Yang Channel of the pair.
4. They demonstrate the important convergences of Qi and Blood in the head and face. The Yin Divergent Channels distribute Qi to the head and face, which supplements the distribution of the

---

[1] Except the San Jiao Divergent Channel which runs downward from the vertex.

Regular Channels. For example, the three Yin Divergent Channels of the hand all pass through the throat and converge with their regular Yang channels at the face. They transport Yin, Essence and Fluids directly to the eyes, nose, mouth, tongue, and ear to nourish and promote the function of the sense organs. This further illustrates the theory that the head and face are where the Qi and Blood converge and collect, providing the theoretical basis for ear, nose, face, scalp, and eye acupuncture.

5. They integrate parts of the body not covered by the Regular Channels in to the channel system. Areas that are not covered by the pathways of the Regular Channels, and organs that are not connected by the Regular Channels, are more securely linked by the Divergent Channels. For example:

   a) The three Yang Divergent Channels of the foot are all connected with the Heart. This establishes the direct connection between the Urinary Bladder and the Heart, the Gall Bladder and the Heart, and the Stomach and the Heart.

   b) The Urinary Bladder Divergent Channel connects with the rectal area and anus, strengthening the connection between that region of the body and Urinary Bladder Regular Channel.

   c) The Kidney Divergent Channel connects with the Dai Channel, the nape, and is further related to the brain through the Urinary Bladder Regular Channel.

   d) The San Jiao Divergent Channel connects with the vertex.

6. They have no points of their own. They share the points of their Regular Channels.

7. According to the Chapter 11, "Divergent Channels," of the Nei Jing Ling Shu (Spiritual Axis), there is no description of Divergent Channel pathology. The Divergent Channels share the same pathology as the Regular Channels.

Summary of the Divergent Channel's Distribution

Channel	Separating	Entering	Emerging	Converging
Urinary Bladder	Popliteal fossa (UB 40)	Sacrum (5 cun above the anus)	Nape (UB 10)	Nape (UB 10)
Kidney	Popliteal fossa (Ki 10)	Same as Urinary Bladder Channel	Nape (UB 10)	Nape (UB 10)
Gall Bladder	Hip (GB 30)	External genitalia	Mandible	Outer Canthus (GB 1)
Liver	Dorsum of the foot (Lv 3)	External genitalia	Mandible	Outer Canthus (GB 1)
Stomach	Front of thigh	St 30 area	Mouth	Inner Canthus (UB 1)
Spleen	Front of thigh	St 30 area (Sp 12)	Throat	Mouth
Small Intestine	Shoulder joint (SI 10)	Axillary fossa	None	None
Heart	Axillary fossa (Ht 1)	Axillary fossa	Face	Inner canthus (UB 1)
San Jiao	Vertex (Du 20 area)	Supraclavicular fossa	None	None
Pericardium	Below axillary fossa (GB 22)	Chest	Retroauricular area	Mastoid process
Large Intestine	Hand	Supraclavicular fossa	Supraclavicular fossa	Throat (LI 18)
Lung	Anterior to axillary fossa (Lu 1)	Chest	Supraclavicular fossa	Throat (LI 18)

The Relationship of Liu He

Liu He means *Six Joining Places*. The twelve Divergent Channels are divided into six Yin and Yang pairs that always circulate together. Each pair joins together at the Separating Point, or at the Converging Point. The Converging Point is also the location where the paired Divergent Channels join the Six Yang Regular Channels of their pair. Clinically, these joining places can be used to treat disorders of the paired channels. They may be used singly or in combination. Because of their connection with the pairs of Divergent Channels, the Six Yang Regular Channels have a strong controlling influence on all twelve Divergent Channels.

Paired Divergent Channels	Joining Places	Converges with (Regular Channel)
Bladder and Kidney	Popliteal fossa/Nape	Urinary Bladder
Gall Bladder and Liver	External genitalia	Gall Bladder
Stomach and Spleen	St 30 area	Stomach
Heart and Small Intestine	Inner canthus	Small Intestine
San Jiao and Pericardium	Inferior to the mastoid process	San Jiao
Large Intestine and Lung	Supraclavicular fossa and throat	Large Intestine

The Clinical Applications of the Twelve Divergent Channels

The Twelve Divergent Channels have additional areas of distribution and organ connections, which go beyond the pathways of their related Regular Channels. They provide the rationale for applying the points to disorders not directly related to the theory of the Regular Channels. The following are examples.

1. They reinforce the connection between paired organs and channels. A disease affecting a Yang organ or channel can be treated by selecting points from its paired channel, and vice versa. For example, if gall bladder is disordered, Lv 3 can be used, and GB 40 can be used for liver disorders.

2. According to the Liu He (Six Joining Places) Relationship, the points where the channels join can be used to treat disorders of the areas where they converge, and vice versa. For example, UB 10, which is the converging point of the Urinary Bladder and Kidney Divergent Channels, can be used to treat the disorders of both the Urinary Bladder and Kidney organs and channels. UB 40 is used to treat the disorders of the nape and neck, while UB 10 can be used for disorders of the popliteal fossa.

3. The Divergent Channels can be used to treat disorders in areas not covered by the pathways of the Regular Channels. For example, UB 40 and UB 57 can be used for prolapse of the rectum and hemorrhoids. Du 4 can be used for treating leukorrhea (a disorder of the Dai Channel). Insomnia and palpitations (which are disorders of the heart) can be treated by points of the Stomach, Gall Bladder, or Urinary Bladder Channel.

C. The Twelve Tendinomuscular Channels

Characteristics:

1. The Tendinomuscular Channels also share the same name as the Regular Channels of which they are a branch. They supplement the Regular Channels by emphasizing the circulation of Qi and Blood to the muscles, tissues, joints, and the body surface.

2. Each of the Tendinomuscular Channels has its own pathway, which generally follows its Regular Channel's pathway. All Tendinomuscular Channels start in the extremities and go to the trunk, or head and face. Their pathways are wider than the Regular Channels, covering broader areas like a band. They usually do not connect with the Zang Fu organs.

3. Their distribution can be summarized in four words: *Jie* (knot) —The Qi and blood of each Tendinomuscular Channel concentrate at certain areas, generally at large muscles or joints. *Ju* (convergences) —These are places where two or more Tendinomuscular Channels bind together. *San* (dispersion) —The Qi disperses in the large muscles as they divide into smaller muscle groups. *Luo* (connecting) —The Tendinomuscular Channels connect the muscles, tendons, and ligaments to the joints to facilitate articulation. The *Jie* concentrations are especially important. Their locations will be described in detail and will be designated by the term **knot** when the pathways of each individual Tendinomuscular Channels are discussed in later chapters.

4. They are divided into four groups of Yin and Yang pairs that demonstrate a special relationship. The three Yang Tendinomuscular Channels of the Foot all connect at the *face* (zygoma). The three Yin Tendinomuscular Channels of the Foot all connect at the *external genitalia*. The three Yang Tendinomuscular Channels of the Hand all connect at the *corner of the head* (temporofrontal region). The three Yin Tendinomuscular Channels of the Hand all connect at the *diaphragm*. Each of these areas has a strong influence on the three related Tendinomuscular Channels.

5. The functions of the Tendinomuscular Channels can be summarized as follows: a) distribute Qi and Blood to the body surface, b) connect the muscles, tendons, and ligaments to the joints, c) protect the bones, d) link the structures of the body, and e) facilitate articulation and normal movement.

6. The Tendinomuscular Channels have no points of their own.

7. Each of the Tendinomuscular Channels has its own pathology. The symptoms and signs are described in Chapter 13, "Tendinomuscular Channels," of the Nei Jing Ling Shu (Spiritual Axis). They mainly involve pain, spasm, and flaccidity of the muscles, stiffness and restricted movement of the joints, and convulsions.

8. The treatment of Tendinomuscular disorders is based on selection of local points. The primary technique is needling with Warming Method.

Pathology of the Twelve Tendinomuscular Channels

Symptoms and Signs

The description of the pathology of the Tendinomuscular Channels here, and in later chapters is taken from Chapter 13, "Tendinomuscular Channels", of the Nei Jing Ling Shu (Spiritual Axis). The signs and symptoms that indicate Tendinomuscular Channel disorders are pain, spasm, stiffness, contraction and pulling sensations of the muscles, tendons, ligaments, and joints. They also include flaccidity and loosening of the muscles. In addition, impaired movement of any kind may indicate a disorder of the Tendinomuscular Channels. This includes restricted extension and flexion of the knee and elbow, inversion and eversion of the foot, forward and backward bending or rotation of the neck, back and lumbar region, and abduction and adduction of the extremities.

Etiology and Pathology

The following may result in a disorder of the Tendinomuscular Channels. They affect the muscles and joints by causing stagnation of Qi and Blood in the channels and collaterals.

1. The Bi Syndromes — External invasion by pathogenic Wind, Cold, Dampness or Heat.
2. Traumatic injury
3. Muscle strain due to overuse.
4. Muscle tension and contraction due to long term mental and emotional stress.

Clinical Applications of the Twelve Tendinomuscular Channels
1. Selection of points
   a) *Ashi points* are primarily selected for Tendinomuscular disorders.
   b) Clinically, we select a combination of local, distal, and adjacent points.
   c) In acute conditions, distal points are used first. This enables the patient to move the affected area while needles are being manipulated, and avoids exacerbating local swelling and bruising.

d) *Miu Ci* method is often used for acute sprain or injury. The name means *treating the corresponding area of the opposite side,* as described in the chart below:

Symptomatic Area	Corresponding Area
Shoulder	Hip
Elbow	Knee
Wrist	Ankle
Hand/Fingers	Foot/Toes
Lumbar/Back	Abdomen/Chest
Neck	Shao Yang, Tai Yang or Yang Ming Channel of Hand and Foot

The appropriate point for Miu Ci technique is selected by first determining which channel or channels are involved. For example, if the tenderest point of an ankle sprain is GB 40, injury of the Shao Yang Tendinomuscular Channel of Foot is indicated. The contralateral corresponding point at the wrist on the Shao Yang Channel of the Hand should be selected, in this case SJ 4. In order to break through the stagnation it is important to constantly move the affected joint while stimulating the point.

2. Methods of Treatment
   a) Acupuncture
* *Fan Zhen Ji Ci*. Ci means puncturing; Fan Zhen Ji Ci means "fire needle with quick insertion and rapid removal." A thick needle (26 - 32 gauge) is heated over a flame until white hot from root to tip. It is then inserted and immediately removed. This technique is used for stubborn Bi syndrome with pain, swelling and joint deformity due to intermingled stagnation of Cold, Damp, Phlegm, Qi, and Blood.
* *Warming Method*. A large piece cut from a moxa stick is put on the handle of a needle and ignited. The heat penetrates through the needle into the point.

Acupuncture is applied with different methods according to the type of Bi Syndrome. The following methods are described in the Nei Jing:

Indication	Technique	Method of application
Ji Bi (Muscle Bi Syndrome)	Fu Ci (Superficial Ci)	Shallow and oblique insertion, 30°- 45° from the edge of the affected area toward the center. This technique is mainly used when superficial muscles are affected.
	He Gu Ci (Chicken Feet Ci)	One needle is inserted perpendicularly in the middle of the affected muscle, then two others are inserted on either side with their tips pointed obliquely toward the middle. This technique is mainly used when deep muscles are affected.
	Pan Geeing Ci (Two needles in a painful area Ci)	One needle is inserted perpendicularly in the middle of the affected area, another is inserted obliquely from the side. This technique is mainly for chronic Muscle Bi Syndrome.
Jing Bi (Tendon and Ligament Bi Syndrome)	Guan Ci (Joint Ci)	Rapidly insert a needle into joints or the extremities for disorder of joints and tendons. Care should be exercised so as not to touch the tendon or cause bleeding. This technique is especially useful for knee and other joint pain.
	Hui Ci (Tendon Ci)	Select points on each end of the affected tendon or muscle on contralaterally. Once inserted, rotate the needles, shake the needles up and down and side to side. This technique is mainly for releasing spasms of muscles and tendons.

Indication	Technique	Method of application
Gu Bi (Bone and Joints Bi Syndrome)	Duan Ci (Bone Ci)	Once the needle is inserted to a shallow level, move to a deep level until close to the bone or joint. Use lifting and thrusting method for deep level Bi Syndrome involving the bones and joints.
	Shu Ci (Deep Ci)	This technique requires quick insertion to and quick withdrawal from the deep level of the affected bone or joint.
Wandering Bi	Bao Ci (Leopard Ci)	Find the most tender spot and a insert needle. Search for another tender spot, remove the previous needle and reinsert.[1] Repeat until all tender spots are treated. The purpose is to drive the pathogen out of the body. Start from the tender spots on the upper body, then move to the lower body.
Cold Bi	Qi Ci (Three needles in a painful area Ci)	Three needles are inserted deeply into the affected area. Insertion can be linear or triangular, either perpendicular or oblique. This technique is used for deep level muscle disorders.
	Yang Ci (Five needles in a painful area Ci)	Insert one needle in the center of the affected area, then four needles around the middle needle obliquely toward the center. This technique is for shallow level muscle disorder.
Hot Bi	Shu Ci (Quick Ci)	This technique requires quick insertion and quick withdrawal using very few needles. It treats Bi syndrome with swelling, redness, and pain

2. Methods of Treatment (continued)

   b) Moxibustion: Direct and indirect moxibustion are both applicable.
   c) Warming methods including hot packs, TDP lamp, and infrared.
   d) Other methods include cupping, electric simulators, Seven Star Needles, and bleeding method, which are often used in combination with acupuncture and moxibustion.

D. Twelve Cutaneous Regions

Characteristics:

1. They share the same name as the regular channel of which they are a branch. They supplement the Regular Channels, emphasizing the circulation of Qi and Blood to the skin and tissues of the body surface.
2. Their distribution follows the course of the Regular Channels on the body surface, covering a wider area than the Regular Channels. They do not distribute interiorly.
3. Their functions are to circulate Qi and Blood, especially the Wei (Defensive) Qi to body surface, regulate the function of the skin and pores, and strengthen the body's immunity. These functions are directly related to the Lung Qi because the Lung is related to the Wei (Defensive) Qi and the skin. External pathogens can enter the body through the Cutaneous Regions.
4. In Chapter 56, "Discussion of Cutaneous Regions," of the Nei Jing Su Wen (Plain Questions), there is no description of pathology for the Cutaneous Regions. Clinically, skin disorders, such as rashes, discolorations, or growths, may indicate a disorder of a Cutaneous Region's related channel and organ.

---

[1] This is the traditional method. Due to current constraints on reusing needles and concerns for autoinfection, additional sterilized needles can be used.

5. The Cutaneous Regions do not have points of their own.
6. The treatment methods for the Cutaneous Regions include shallow and transverse needle insertion, Gua Sha, Seven Star Needles, intradermal needles, cupping, and moxibustion.

The Eight Extraordinary Channels

Characteristics
The Eight Extraordinary Channels have both similar and dissimilar characteristics from those of the Twelve Channel System.
1. Each channels has its own name. They are the Du, Ren, Chong, Dai, Yin Wei, Yang Wei, Yin Qiao and Yang Qiao Channels.
2. They are distributed all over the body except on the upper extremities. Their courses and distributions must be learned separately from the Regular Channels. They run from the extremities to the trunk and head, or vice versa, or transversely around the trunk.
3. Their functions are storing the Qi and Blood, and distributing them to the Twelve Channel System. Like lakes and reservoirs for storing surplus water, the Eight Extraordinary Channels store the Qi and Blood, returning them to the Twelve Channel system when needed.
4. They control and supplement the Twelve Channel System, grouping the Regular Channels together, and providing a regulating function. For instance, the Du Channel governs all the Yang channels, the Ren Channel controls all the Yin Channels, and the Chong Channel regulates all twelve regular channels.
5. Each of the Eight Extra Channels has its own pathology.
6. Of the Eight Extra Channels, only the Ren and Du Channels have points of their own. The other six Extraordinary Channels share the points of the other fourteen channels.

General Functions of the Eight Extraordinary Channels

Du Channel	*Sea of Yang Qi.* It governs all the Yang Channels and is related to the function of the brain, and spinal column.
Ren Channel	*Sea of Yin Qi.* It controls all the Yin Channels and is related to gynecological, obstetrical, and urogenital functions.
Chong Channel	*Sea of Blood.* It controls the twelve channels and is related to gynecological and blood functions.
Dai Channel	Binds all the channels together. It is related to leukorrhea and the function of the lower extremities.
Yin Qiao and Yang Qiao	Together they maintain the proper cycle of sleep, controlling the opening and closing of the eyes. They also control the movement and balance of the lower extremities.
Yin Wei and Yang Wei	Together they balance the Yin and Yang aspects of the four extremities. Yang Wei dominates the exterior, Yin Wei dominates the interior.

The Luo Collateral System

Key Points
- The Luo Collaterals are branches of the Regular Channels. They are comprised of the of Sixteen Major Luo Collaterals and the Small Luo Collaterals. The Small Luo Collaterals are divided into the Minute, Blood, Grandson, and Superficial Luo Collaterals.

- Together with the Channel System they form a network to integrate the entire body and distribute Qi and Blood, especially to the surface.
- The Sixteen Major Luo Collaterals take a leading role in controlling and mastering all the Luo Collaterals of the body.
- Each of the Sixteen Luo Collaterals has its own pathology. Pathogenic factors generally enter the body through the Superficial Luo Collaterals and stagnation of Qi and Blood in the channels and the organs may be reflected and observed in the Blood Luo Collaterals.
- When treating disorders of the Luo Collaterals, shallow acupuncture, moxibustion, and cupping are generally applied. Pricking method, Seven Star Needles, and bleeding method can also be applied to remove stagnation from the collaterals.

The Sixteen Major Luo Collaterals

Characteristics

1. There are Sixteen Major Luo Collaterals. They share the name of the Regular and Extraordinary Channels of which they are a branch. The Twelve Regular Channels each have a Major Luo Collateral. Of the Eight Extraordinary Channels, only the Ren and Du Channels have a Major Luo Collateral. Spleen and Stomach Channels each have an extra Major Luo Collateral.
2. Each Major Luo Collateral has a specific point from which it separates from the its Regular Channel called a *Luo (Connecting) Point*.
3. Their distribution is mainly on the surface of the body. The Luo Collaterals of the Yin Channels are connected with the Yang Channels, and vice versa. Many of them have their own pathways.
4. The function of the Luo Collaterals is to reinforce the connection between the paired Regular and Extraordinary channels on the body surface. They usually do not have a connection to the internal organs.
5. According to Chapter 10, "Chapter of Channels," of Nei Jing Ling Shu (Spiritual Axis), each of the Sixteen Luo Collaterals has its own pathology.

Clinical Applications

The Sixteen Luo (Connecting) points are mainly used to treat:

1. Disorders of their internally/externally related channels. For example Sp 4 can be used to treat stomach pain, and St 40 can be used to treat Spleen disorders such as diarrhea, abdominal distention, and poor appetite.
2. Luo Collateral disorders. The symptoms and signs of the Luo Collaterals are described in Chapter 10, "Chapter of Channels," of Nei Jing Ling Shu (Spiritual Axis). They are usually characterized as either excess, deficiency, or rebellion of Qi in the Luo Collateral. For example, when Qi is in excess in the Pericardium Channel it may result in cardiac pain, angina pectoris, and chest pain. When Qi is deficient in the Pericardium Channel, it may result in restlessness and irritability. In either case, the Luo (Connecting) point, Pc 6, may be used for treatment.
3. Disorders of the Luo Collaterals' distribution. For example, Ht 5 treats stuffiness of the chest in cases of excess, and aphasia in those of deficiency. Due to the Luo Collateral's connection to the eye, it can also be used to treat disorders of the eye.
4. Whole body disorders. The two Major Luo Collaterals, Sp 21 and St 18, are used for disorders of the whole body, as well as their own specific distribution.

IV. The Channel System's Relationship with the Organs and Other Body Structures

The following is a summary of the connection between the Channel System's pathways and the internal organs:

1. **The Lung** is connected by the Lung Regular Channel, the Lung Divergent Channel, the Large Intestine Regular Channel, the Large Intestine Divergent Channels, the Heart Regular Channel, the Kidney Regular Channel, the Liver Regular Channel, and the Ren Channel.

2. **The Large Intestine** is connected by the Large Intestine Regular Channel, the Large Intestine Divergent Channel, the Stomach Regular Channel, the Lung Regular Channel, and the Spleen Luo Collateral.

3. **The Stomach** is connected by the Stomach Regular Channel, the Stomach Divergent Channel, the Large Intestine Regular Channel, the Small Intestine Regular Channel, the Spleen Regular Channel, the Spleen Divergent Channel, the Spleen Luo Collateral, the Liver Regular Channel, and the Chong Channel.

4. **The Spleen** is connected by the Spleen Regular Channel, the Spleen Divergent Channel, the Stomach Regular Channel, and the Stomach Divergent Channel.

5. **The Heart** is connected by the Heart Regular Channel, the Heart Divergent Channel, the Heart Luo Collateral, the Small Intestine Regular Channel, the Stomach Divergent Channel, the Spleen Regular Channel, the Spleen Divergent Channel, the Gall Bladder Divergent Channel, the Urinary Bladder Divergent Channel, the Du Channel, and the Chong Channel.

6. **The Small Intestine** is connected by the Small Intestine Regular Channel, the Small Intestine Divergent Channel, the Stomach Regular Channel, and the Heart Regular Channel.

7. **The Urinary Bladder** is connected by the Urinary Bladder Regular Channel, Urinary Bladder Divergent Channel, and the Kidney Regular Channel.

8. **The Kidney** is connected by the Kidney Regular Channel, the Kidney Divergent Channel, the Urinary Bladder Regular Channel, the Du Channel, the Ren Channel, and the Chong Channel.

9. **The Pericardium** is connected by the Pericardium Regular Channel, the San Jiao Regular Channel, and the Kidney Regular Channel.

10. **The San Jiao** is connected by the San Jiao Regular Channel, the San Jiao Divergent Channel, the Pericardium Regular Channel, and the Pericardium Divergent Channel.

11. **The Gall Bladder** is connected by the Gall Bladder Regular Channel, the Gall Bladder Divergent Channel, and the Liver Regular Channel.

12. **The Liver** is connected by the Liver Regular Channel, the Gall Bladder Regular Channel, the Gall Bladder Divergent Channel, and the Kidney Regular Channel.

The following is the summary of the Channel System's connections to the sense organs and other body structures.

1. **The eye (system).** The Stomach Regular Channel, the Stomach Divergent Channel, the Stomach Tendinomuscular Channel, the Heart Regular Channel, the Heart Luo Collateral, the Small Intestine Regular Channel, the Small Intestine Tendinomuscular Channel, the Urinary Bladder Regular Channel, the Urinary Bladder Tendinomuscular Channel, the San Jiao Regular Channel, the San Jiao Tendinomuscular Channel, the Gall Bladder Regular Channel, the Gall Bladder Divergent Channel, the Gall Bladder Tendinomuscular Channel, the Liver Regular Channel, the Ren Channel, and the Du Channel connect with the eye system.

2. **The inner canthus.** The Stomach Regular Channel, the Heart Divergent Channel, the Small Intestine Regular Channel, the Urinary Bladder Regular Channel, the Yang Qiao Channel, and the Yin Qiao Channel connect with the inner canthus.

3. **The outer canthus.** The Small Intestine Regular Channel, the Small Intestine Tendinomuscular Channel, the San Jiao Regular Channel, the San Jiao Tendinomuscular Channel, the Gall Bladder Regular Channel, the Gall Bladder Divergent Channel, and the Gall Bladder Tendinomuscular Channel connect with the outer canthus.

4. **The ear.** The Large Intestine Luo Collateral, the Small Intestine Regular Channel, the Small Intestine Tendinomuscular Channel, the San Jiao Regular Channel, and the Gall Bladder Regular Channel connect with the ear.

5. **The nose and nasopharynx.** The Large Intestine Regular Channel, the Stomach Regular Channel, the Stomach Divergent Channel, the Stomach Tendinomuscular Channel, the Urinary Bladder Tendinomuscular Channel, the Gall Bladder Tendinomuscular Channel, the Liver Regular Channel, the Du Channel, and the Chong Channel connect with the nose and nasopharynx.

6. **The tongue.** The Spleen Regular Channel, the Spleen Divergent Channel, the Heart Luo Collateral, the Urinary Bladder Tendinomuscular Channel, the Kidney Regular Channel, the Kidney Divergent Channel, and the San Jiao Tendinomuscular Channel connect with the tongue.

7. **The lips.** The Large Intestine Regular Channel, the Stomach Regular Channel, the Liver Regular Channel, the Ren Channel, and the Du Channel connect with the lips.

8. **The mouth.** The Stomach Regular channel, the Stomach Divergent Channel, the Stomach Tendinomuscular Channel, and the Gall Bladder Divergent Channel connect with the mouth.

9. **The teeth and gums** The Large Intestine Regular Channel, the Large Intestine Luo Collateral, and the Stomach Regular Channel connect with the teeth and gums.

10. **The throat.** The Lung Divergent Channel, the Large Intestine Divergent Channel, the Large Intestine Regular Channel, the Stomach Regular Channel, the Stomach Divergent Channel, the Stomach Luo Collateral, the Spleen Divergent Channel, the Heart Regular Channel, the Liver Regular Channel, the Ren Channel, the Du Channel, and the Yin Wei Channel connects with the throat.

11. **The Ho Yin (anus).** The Kidney Regular Channel, Urinary Bladder Divergent Channel, Du Channel, Ren Channel, and Chong Channel connect with the Ho Yin.

12. **The Qian Yin (urethra and vagina).** The Liver Regular, Divergent, Tendinomuscular Channel, the Liver Luo Collateral, Gall Bladder Divergent Channel, Du Channel, and the Ren Channel connect with the Qian Yin.

13. **The external genitalia.** The Liver Regular Channel, the Liver Divergent Channel, the Liver Tendinomuscular Channel, the Liver Luo Collateral, the Gall Bladder Divergent Channel, the Stomach Tendinomuscular Channel, Spleen Tendinomuscular Channel, Kidney Tendinomuscular Channel, the Ren Channel, the Du Channel, and Yin Qiao Channel connect with the external genitalia.

14. **The breast.** The Large Intestine Divergent Channel, the Stomach Regular Channel, the Stomach Tendinomuscular Channel, the Pericardium Regular Channel, the Pericardium Tendinomuscular Channel, and the Heart Tendinomuscular Channel connect with the breast.

15. **The spine.** The Du Channel, the Ren Channel, the Spleen Tendinomuscular Channel, the Kidney Regular Channel, the Kidney Divergent Channel, the Kidney Luo Collateral, the Chong Channel, and the Dai Channel connect with the spine.

16. **The brain.** The Du Channel, the Urinary Bladder Regular Channel, the Kidney Divergent Channel, the Yang Qiao Channel, the Yin Qiao Channel, and the Liver Regular Channel connect with the brain.

17. **The uterus.** The Ren Channel, the Du Channel, the Chong Channel, and the Kidney Regular Channel connect with the uterus.

18. **The umbilicus.** The Spleen Tendinomuscular Channel, the Heart Tendinomuscular Channel, the Du Channel, and the Ren Channel connect with the umbilicus.

19. **The temporofrontal region (corner of the head).** The Stomach Regular Channel, the Gall Bladder Regular Channel, the Gall Bladder Tendinomuscular Channel, the Large Intestine Tendinomuscular Channel, the Small Intestine Tendinomuscular Channel, and the San Jiao Tendinomuscular Channel connect with the temporofrontal region.

The Twelve Channel System

1. The Lung Channel of Hand - Tai Yin
手 太 陰 肺 經

Key Points
- The Lung Channel starts in the chest (Lu 1).
- The channel ends at the index finger (connects with the Large Intestine Channel at LI 1).
- It distributes mainly on the medioanterior aspect of the upper extremities.
- It connects with the lung and the large Intestine.
- There are 11 points altogether.

The Pathway of the Lung Regular Channel[1]

Internal Pathway
The Lung Regular Channel begins in the Middle Jiao (Ren 12), the source of Qi and Blood. From the Middle Jiao, the channel flows downward and directly connects with the large intestine, then returns to the stomach. After leaving the stomach, it passes through the cardiac orifice, through the diaphragm, and into the Lungs (its pertaining organ). It emerges from the chest at Ren 22, where it connects with the throat[2].

External Pathway
From the throat area the Regular Channel travels to the superolateral aspect of the chest (Lu 1), then down the arm, distributing on the medioanterior aspect. When it reaches the styloid process of the radius, it divides. One branch follows the border of the thenar eminence and ends at the radial side of the thumb (Lu 11). The other goes to the radial side of the index finger, where it connects with the Large Intestine Regular Channel (LI 1).

The Associated Organs and Points

Pertains to	Connects with	Associated With	Intersecting Points
Lung	Large intestine	Stomach, Lung system (upper respiratory tract, bronchi, pharynx, larynx, other throat structures)	None

Physiology

The Lung dominates the Qi of the whole body, and the Lung Channel is responsible for the circulation of Qi to the entire body, and performs the following functions:

---

[1] The description of the pathways of the regular channels are taken from Chapter 10, "Chapter of Channels", of the Nei Jing Ling Shu (Spiritual Axis).

[2] The throat in this context includes the larynx, pharynx and vocal cords.

16

1. *Circulate Qi.* It is especially important for circulating the Wei (Defensive) Qi, to the body surface, and strengthen the body's resistance to external attack, so that the normal body temperature and perspiration can be maintained.
2. *Promote the circulation of Qi in the chest, nourishing and harmonizing the function of the lung and heart.*
3. *Regulate the ascending and descending of Qi.* The descending function of Lung Qi complements the ascending function of Liver Qi. The two together harmonizes the movement of Qi, prevent excesses, and assisting the other organs to maintain their proper direction of Qi circulation.
4. *Regulate Body Fluid circulation.* This including the volume and color of urine.
5. *Spread the Qi and Lift the Spirit.* For this reason, the Lung Regular Channel is effective for mental and emotional difficulties.
6. The Lung Regular Channel is connected to the stomach, large intestine, throat, shoulder, upper back, arms, thenar eminence, and thumb. The points of the Lung Channel are effective for disorders of all these areas.

Pathology

Channel Pathology from the Nei Jing[1]

Lung channel dominates the disorders of the lungs. When Lung Qi is disturbed, there will be rebellious Qi, cough, asthma, chest fullness, restlessness, thirst, pain on the medial aspect of the arm, and hot palms. There may also be **Bi Jue Syndrome**[2] which includes distention and fullness of the chest, constant asthmatic cough, pain in the supraclavicular fossa, and the gesture of holding the chest (with folded arms). *Excess of Qi* in the channel will cause shoulder and back pain, aversion to cold with sweating due to Wind attack, and frequent urination with decreased volume. *Deficiency of Qi* will cause shoulder and back pain, aversion to cold, shortness of breath, and a change in the color of urine.

Summary of Channel Pathology

The symptom complexes of channel pathology presented below are gathered from several sources. The primary symptoms are from chapter 10, "Chapter of Channels," of the Nei Jing Ling Shu (Spiritual Axis). Additional symptoms come from other chapters of the Nei Jing, both the Ling Shu (Spiritual Axis) and Su Wen (Plain Questions), and from later medical classics.

Dominates Disorders of	Lung
Channel Disorder	• <u>Exterior Syndrome</u>: aversion to cold, fever with or without sweating, nasal obstruction, headache. • <u>Allergic Symptoms</u>: frequent sneezing, watering and itching of the eyes, nose and throat. • <u>Disorders of the Nose and Throat</u>: rhinitis, sinusitis, swelling, and pain of the throat. • <u>Channel Obstruction</u>: pain, hot, cold, or other abnormal sensation in supraclavicular fossa, chest, upper back, shoulder, elbow, arm, wrist, and thumb.

---

[1] The pathology of the regular channels is taken from Chapter 10, "Chapter of Channels", of the Nei Jing Ling Shu (Spiritual Axis).

[2] Bi Jue Syndrome - Bi means the arm. The original meaning of Jue is cold hands and feet. In this particular case, Jue means an abnormal condition.

Summary of Channel Pathology (continued)

Organ Disorder	• <u>Lung system</u>: cough, asthma, shortness of breath, sputum, hemoptysis, weak and low voice, fatigue, frequent colds. • <u>Chest and heart</u>: chest pain and a stifling sensation, palpitations, restlessness. • <u>Body Fluids</u>: yellow urine, unsmooth, frequent urination, incontinence, edema. • <u>Large intestine</u>: abdominal fullness and distention, loose stools, diarrhea, constipation. • <u>Stomach</u>: distending pain, burning sensation in the epigastric region or behind the sternum

The Clinical Applications

The points of Lung Channel are mainly used for disorders of the lung, chest, throat, and body fluids, as well as those occurring along the Lung Channel distribution.

Category	Examples of Symptoms and Signs	Key points in order of importance[1]	Combinations with points from other channels.
Exterior Syndrome	• <u>Wind Cold or Wind Heat</u> Common cold, influenza. • <u>Allergy</u>: especially with sneezing, itching throat and nose.	Lu 7, 5, 11 Lu 7, 5, 9	LI 4, LI 11, SJ 5, UB 12, GB 20 Du 14, UB 12, GB 20, St 36
Immuno-deficiency	• <u>Wei (Nutritive) Qi deficiency</u>: frequent colds, low energy. • <u>Whole body Qi deficiency</u>: cold hand and feet, low energy, chronic fatigue syndrome, chronic diseases.	Lu 9, 7, 8 Lu 9, 7	St 36, Du 12, UB 13, UB 23, UB 43 Ren 6, St 36, Du 14, UB 13, UB 23, UB 43
Respiratory Disorders	• Cough • Asthma • Breathing difficulties	Lu 5, 8, 7, 6, 1, 9 Lu 6, 5, 10, 9 Lu 5, 8, 7, 1	St 40, 41, Ki 6, LI 4 Ren 17, Dingchuan Ren 17, Du 12, Pc 6, Ki 7, St 40
Nose and Throat Disorders	• Nasal obstruction, runny nose, rhinitis, sinusitis, • Dry throat, pharyngitis, laryngitis, tonsillitis	Lu 7, 10 Lu 10, 7, 11	LI 4, LI 11, SJ 5, GB 40, UB 7, UB 58 LI 1, LI 4, SJ 2, St 44, Ki 6, UB 10
Body Fluids and Urinary Disorders	• Edema • Enuresis • Retention of urine, difficult urination	Lu 7, 5 Lu 7 Lu 7, 5	Sp 9, St 40, Ren 9, UB 13, UB 23 Ren 4, Du 4, UB 23 Ren 3, UB 28, Sp 6, Sp 9, Lv 5

---

[1] Point prescriptions are based on the classical sources and personal experience unless otherwise noted.

The Clinical Applications (continued)

Category	Examples of Symptoms and Signs	Key points in order of importance	Combinations with points from other channels.
Large Intestine Disorders	• Diarrhea • Constipation • Hemorrhoids	Lu 7 Lu 7, 10 Lu 6	LI 11, LI 4, St 25, St 37, St 36 LI 11, St 39, Sp 15, SJ 6, Ki 6 UB 57, Er Bai, UB 35
Stomach Disorders	• Hyperacidity • Pain • Retention of phlegm fluid in the stomach	Lu 5, 10 Lu 6, 7 Lu 1, 5, 7, 9	St 44, Ren 13, UB 44, Lv 2 Pc 6, St 36, Ren 10, St 21 St 40, Sp 3, Pc 6, UB 20, UB 21
Headache	• <u>Frontal</u>: sinus, common cold, indigestion. • <u>Temporal</u>: headache, migraine. • <u>Occipital</u>: common cold, stress, PMS, menstrual disorders.	Lu 7 Lu 7 Lu 7	LI 4, LI 11, St 43 SJ 3, SJ 5, GB 41, GB 31, GB 26 SI 3, UB 62, 65, Sp 4, Lv 3
Emotional and Mental Disorders	• Sighing, mental stress, restlessness, chest stuffiness, breathing difficulties, shallow breathing, sadness, weeping, grief, anxiety.	Lu 7, 2, 3	Ht 7, Pc 6, Ren 17, Ki 4, SJ 3, St 9, UB 42, Sky Window points[1]
Channel Disorders	• Bi Syndrome of the shoulder, arm, wrist and thumb. • Shoulder, neck and upper back pain, may be due to either mental and physical stress.	Lu 7, 1, 5 Lu 7, 9, 2	Choose local points from the affected channels. Distal points are: St 38, Sp 9, GB 34, GB 39, St 39, LI 4, LI 10, SI 3, SI 11, SJ 5

The Lung Divergent Channel[2]

Pathway

The Lung Divergent Channel separates from the Lung Regular Channel at the anterior aspect of the axillary fossa (Lu 1 area). From there, it enters the chest, then connects with the lung, then with the large intestine. It then goes back upward, emerges at the supraclavicular fossa, and connects with the throat (LI 18 area), where it converges with the Large Intestine Regular Channel.

Separates from	Anterior to the axillary fossa (Lu 1 area)
Enters the body cavity at	Chest
Connects with	Lung, large intestine, throat
Emerges from	Supraclavicular fossa
Converges with the Large Intestine Regular Channel at	Throat (LI 18 area)

---

[1] This refers to the points that have the word "Tian" (which means heaven) in their name. They are often used to treat the disorders of the head and face, and are also effective for releasing mental and emotional stress. There are sixteen points altogether: Lu 3, LI 17, St 25, Sp 18, SI 11, SI 16, SI 17, UB 7, UB 10, Pc 1, Pc 2, SJ 15, SJ 16, SJ 10, GB 9, and Ren 22. Some texts also list St 9 as a Sky Window point.

[2] The description of the pathways of the divergent channels are taken from Chapter 11, "Divergent Channels", of the Nei Jing Ling Shu (Spiritual Axis).

Clinical Applications

The Lung Divergent Channel further reinforces the relationship between the lung and large intestine organs that was established by the Lung Regular Channel. This provides additional theoretical basis for treating the disorders of its paired channel.

For example, LI 11 can be used for treating cough, asthma, and chest pain, while Lu 10 can be used for constipation and diarrhea.

The Divergent Channel demonstrates an additional link between the Lung Channel and the throat, especially the LI 18 area (its Converging Point). This further supports the choice of Lung points (such as Lu 10 and Lu 11) for disorders of the throat such as tonsillitis, pharyngitis, and laryngitis, and well as disorders of the vocal cords and thyroid.

The *Converging Point (LI 18)* has an expanded area of energetic influence. Its application is not confined to the local area or the Large Intestine Channel, but extends to disorders of the Lung Channel. It may be used for arm pain, carpal tunnel syndrome, cough, asthma, breathlessness, and Plum Pit Qi. The combination of the Converging Point and Separating Point (Lu 1) can also be used to treat disorders of both Lung and Large Intestine Channels.

The Lung Tendinomuscular Channel[1]

- Starts from: Thumb (Lu 11)
- Ends at: Hypochondriac region
- Qi accumulates at: Thenar eminence, elbow, shoulder, supraclavicular fossa and chest; distributes in the diaphragm and hypochondriac region.

Pathway

The Lung Tendinomuscular Channel follows the Regular Channel to the thenar eminence, where it **knots**[2]. From there, it then goes to the elbow joint where it **knots** again, then up to and through the area inferior to the axillary fossa. It continues up to, and **knots** at the supraclavicular fossa.

There are two branches that emerge from the supraclavicular fossa. One goes to the anterior aspect of the shoulder where it **knots**. The other enters, and **knots** in the chest, distributes in the intercostal spaces, and goes down through the diaphragm, where the two sides of the channel meet and distribute along the diaphragm and hypochondriac region.

Pathology[3]

1. Stiffness, pulling, spasm, and pain along the course of the Tendinomuscular Channel.
2. *Xi Fen* - Spasm and pain of the chest and hypochondria region. In severe cases, there may be hematemesis.

Clinical Applications

The main application of the Lung Tendinomuscular Channel is Bi Syndrome along the Lung Channel's distribution. It can be used for pain and spasm of the thumb, radial side of the wrist, lateral elbow, anterior aspect of the shoulder, and upper back.

The Tendinomuscular Channel has additional areas of distribution not covered by the Regular Channel. This additional distribution expands the use of Lung Channel points to disorders of the chest and the intercostal, and hypochondriac regions. For example Lu 7, Lu 5, and Lu 6 are often used in

---

[1] The description of the pathways of the tendinomuscular channels are taken from Chapter 13, "Tendinomuscular Channels", of the Nei Jing Ling Shu (Spiritual Axis).

[2] For an explanation of the significance of the *Jie (knots)* of the Tendinomuscular Channels, please refer to the Chapter of the Theory of the Twelve Channels, Section III. Characteristics of the Channel System, Subsection C. The Tendinomuscular Channels.

[3] The description of the pathology of the tendinomuscular channels are taken from Chapter 13, "Tendinomuscular Channels", of the Nei Jing Ling Shu (Spiritual Axis).

combination with Pc 6, St 40, SJ 5, GB 34, and Ren 17, for intercostal neuralgia and costal chondritis. Lu 7 and Lu 5 can be used in combination with LI 10, St 40, Lv 3, UB 17, and Ren 13 for disorders of the breast and diaphragm, including fibrocystic breast disease, hiccup and hiatal hernia,

The Luo Collateral of Lung Channel[1]

Luo point: Lu 7
Distribution: After separating from Lung Channel it disperses into the palm and thenar eminence.
Connection: Palm, thenar eminence, Large Intestine Channel.

Pathology
Excess: Burning pain, hot sensation in the palms and wrists.
Deficiency: Yawning, shortness of breath, frequent urination, enuresis.

Clinical Applications
Lu 7 covers a wide range of applications. This is because in addition to being the Luo (Connecting) point, it also the Confluent point of the Ren Channel. The following is a summary of its Luo (Connecting) applications.

Channel Disorders
Lu 7 is used for hot palms due to Lung Yin deficiency or heat in the Lung Channel. It is also used for traumatic wrist pain and carpal tunnel syndrome, as well as thumb and finger arthritis. Points used in combination with Lu 7 are: Pc 6, Pc 7, SI 4, and GB 34.

Organ Disorders
1. Shortness of Breath and Yawning:
Deficiency Case: This may be due to either Lung Qi or Spleen Qi deficiency. It may also be accompanied by Phlegm fluid retention, as a complication. The Luo (Connecting) point is effective in either case. Points used in combination with Lu 7 are: Lu 9, Sp 3, St 40, and Ren 6.
Excess Case: Breathing may be rapid, and shallow breathing to the extent that it is no deeper than the uppermost area of the chest. This is caused by restrained Lung Qi or to Spleen Qi, which is unable to ascend. This condition is caused by emotional disturbances such as sadness, grief, depression, anxiety and worry. Lu 7 is often used in combination with: UB 42.[2]
2. Frequent Urination
Excess Case: Lu 7 can be effectively used for a) Damp Heat in the Lower Jiao which causes frequent, painful, unsmooth, and yellow urination, and b) stressful situations which may cause frequent urination with urgency. In either case, Lu 7 is used in combination with: Sp 6, Lv 3, St 28, and Lv 5.
Deficiency Case: Lu 7 is also indicated for frequent, clear urination with large volume, due to deficiency of Lung and Kidney Qi, which is then unable to retain the urine. Points used in combination with Lu 7 are: Ki 3, UB 23, St 36, and Du 4.
3. Enuresis
Enuresis occurs mainly in children. Lu 7 can be used for any type of enuresis. Intradermal needles and seed therapy are often used in these cases.

---

[1] The description of the pathways of the luo collaterals are taken from Chapter 10, "Chapter of Channels", of the Nei Jing Ling Shu (Spiritual Axis).

[2] UB 42 is the "residence of corporeal soul" point.

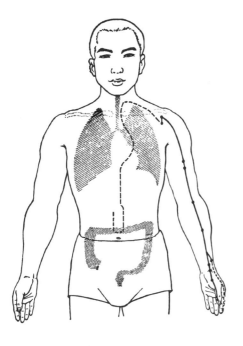

Lung Regular Channel

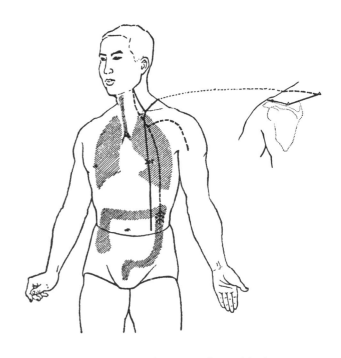

Lung Divergent Channel (---)
LI Divergent Channel (—)

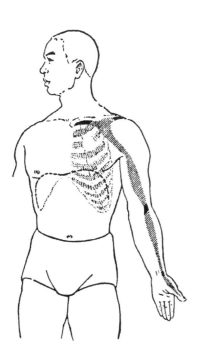

Lung Tendinomuscular Channel

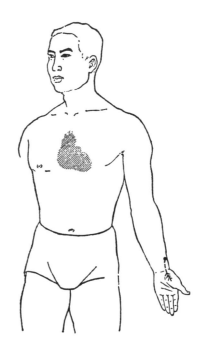

Lung Collateral

The Lung Channel of Hand-Taiyin
手太陰肺經系統分布圖

2. The Large Intestine Channel of Hand - Yang Ming
手 陽 明 大 腸 經

Key Points
- The Large Intestine Channel starts at the radial side of the index finger (LI 1).
- The Channel ends at sides of the ala nasi (LI 20) where it connects with the Stomach Channel.
- It distributes mainly on the lateroanterior aspect of the upper extremities, neck, and face.
- It connects with the large intestine and lung.
- There are 20 points altogether.

The Pathway of the Large Intestine Regular Channel

External Pathway
From LI 1, the Large Intestine Channel flows up the index finger, between the first and second metacarpal bones, then to the wrist joint. From there, it goes up the arm to the lateral aspect of the elbow, to the depression on the lateroanterior aspect of the shoulder near the acromioclavicular joint, then to the upper back (intersects SI 12 and Du 14[1]). From the upper back, it travels to the supraclavicular fossa, where the channel bifurcates. One branch goes internally, entering the chest cavity to begin the internal pathway. The other runs along the side of the neck, through the cheek, into the lower gum. It circles the lips, crossing over from right to left, and from left to right (intersects St 4, Du 26), and ends at the ala nasi (LI 20).

Internal Pathway
From the supraclavicular fossa, the channel enters the body cavity, connecting with the lung. It then passes through the diaphragm and further to the St 25 area, from which it connects with the large intestine. According to Chapter 4, "Pathogenic Qi and Zang Fu", of the Nei Jing Ling Shu (Spiritual Axis), there is a branch from the large intestine organ which descends to St 37, the Lower He (Sea) point of Large Intestine Channel.

The Associated Organs and Points

Pertains to	Connects with	Associated With	Intersecting Points
Large intestine	Lung	Stomach, gums, nose, throat[2]	SI 12, Du 14, St 4, Du 26

Physiology

The Large Intestine Channel has the following functions:
1. *Distribute Qi to the head and face and normalize the function of its associated sense organs and the throat.* Symptoms such as obstruction of the nose, runny nose, allergies, frontal headache, toothache, sore throat, and thyroid disorders implicate a disorder of the Large Intestine Channel.
2. *Regulate the Body Fluids.* According to Chapter 10, "Chapter of Channels," of the Nei Jing Ling Shu (Spiritual Axis), the Large Intestine Channel dominates the disorders of body fluids, called *Jin and*

---

[1] All the Yang channels meet at Du 14.

[2] The throat in this context includes the larynx, pharynx, vocal cords, and the thyroid and parathyroid glands

Ye[1]. Lack of, or excessive perspiration, dry eyes and mouth, diarrhea, and edema may implicate a disorder of the Large Intestine Channel.

3. *Circulate Qi to the arm, shoulder, and neck.* Large Intestine Channel points can be used to treat arthritis, tendinitis, muscular pain or atrophy of the hand, wrist, elbow, shoulder and neck.

4. *Maintain normal function of the large intestine.* This includes normal peristalsis, lubrication and regular elimination of the bowels. Symptoms such as constipation, diarrhea and abdominal pain may indicate a disorder of the Large Intestine Channel.

5. *Clear heat from the blood and channels.* The Yang Ming Channels have abundant Qi and Blood. Fever and heat are considered the result of excessive Qi and Blood in the Yang Ming Channels. This excess gives rise to such symptoms as dry mouth, excessive perspiration, yellow urination, constipation, and skin disorders such as pimples, rashes, boils, and carbuncles.

6. *Tonify Qi and Blood.* This channel tonifies and promotes the circulation of Qi and Blood.

Pathology

Channel Pathology from the Nei Jing

The Large Intestine Channel dominates the disorders of Body Fluids. If the Large Intestine Channel is disordered, there will be toothache, swelling of the neck, yellow sclera, dry mouth. The nasal passages may be obstructed or runny. There may be epistaxis. There can also be blockage of the throat and pain of the shoulder, arm, and index finger. When there is *excess Qi* in the channel, there will be heat and swelling along the channel. When there is a *deficiency of Qi* in the channel, there will be shivering due to aversion to cold and difficulty in regaining warmth.

Summary of Channel Pathology

Dominates Disorders of	Body Fluids (Jin and Ye)	
Channel Disorder	• <u>Exterior Syndrome</u>: fever, chills, obstruction of the nose, Yang Ming headache. • <u>Heat Syndrome</u>: fever, hot sensation of the body, sweating, thirst, concentrated, yellow urination. • <u>Head and Face, Sense Organ Disorders</u>: sinusitis, epistaxis, swelling and painful throat, toothache (due to swollen gums), pain and redness of the eyes,[2] swelling of the neck, hyperthyroidism, facial paralysis. • <u>Skin Disorders</u>: swelling, rashes, itching, discoloration, discharge and pain of the skin. • <u>Channel Obstruction</u>: pain, swelling, hot, cold or other abnormal sensation on the hand, arm, shoulder and scapular region, upper back and neck	
Organ Disorder	• <u>Large intestine</u>: abdominal pain, umbilicus area pain, borborygmus, flatulence, diarrhea which may be yellow and sticky, constipation, • <u>Lung</u>: cough, asthma, sputum, chest pain, low energy. • Stomach: epigastric pain, vomiting, belching	
Body Fluid Disorders	• <u>Excess</u>: diarrhea, runny nose, facial edema, sweating • <u>Deficiency</u>: dry mouth and throat, thirst, dry stool, lack of sweating.	

---

[1] Body fluids is called Jin Ye. The Jin is called "thin", like urine, sweat, tears, and saliva. The Ye is more turbid like lubricating fluids, e.g. synovial.

[2] Large Intestine channel connects to the eyes through the Stomach channel.

The Clinical Applications

The points of the Large Intestine Channel are mainly used for treating disorders of the channel, the head and face, and the Body Fluids. Because the three Yang channels of the hand start from the hand and go to the face, they mainly treat disorders along their channel's distribution. Their related Fu organ disorders are mainly treated by the respective Lower He (Sea) points.

Category	Examples of Symptoms and Signs	Key points in order of importance.	Combinations with points from other channels.
Channel disorders	• Pain, hot and cold sensations, swelling of upper back, scapula, neck, shoulder, elbow, arm and hand.	LI 15, 11, 4, 10	Lu 7, SJ 8, SI 12
Head, face, sense organ disorders	• Headache (mainly Yang Ming) • Toothache • Facial paralysis, trigeminal neuralgia, TMJ Syndrome • Rhinitis, sinusitis • Epistaxis • Redness of the eyes, yellow sclera	LI 4, 3, 11 LI 4, 7, 3 LI 4, 11, 7 LI 4, 11, 20 LI 2, 4, 7 LI 2, 4, 11, 14	Yintang, Lu 7, St 43, St 44, UB 2 St 44, Lu 7, Ki 6 Lu 7, Lv 3, St 37, SJ 3, SJ 5, St 7 Lu 7, St 36, UB 58, St 37 Lu 4, Lu 6, Lu 10, Ki 6 Lv 2, Lv 3, SI 2, GB 37
Throat and neck disorders	• Swollen and painful throat • Vocal cord disorders • Thyroid disorders	LI 1, 2, 4, 18 LI 4, 5, 11, 18 LI 11, 4, 14, 18	Lu 10, Lu 7, SJ 2, SI 17, St 9 Lu 7, Ht 5, St 40 SJ 5, 13, St 40, Ht 5, Pc 5
Exterior Syndrome	• Wind Heat or Wind Cold (common cold, influenza) • Allergy (especially with burning and itching sensation of skin and sense organs)	LI 4, 11 LI 11, 4, 3, 20	Lu 7, SJ 5, UB 12 Lu 7, Du 14, St 36, GB 20
Body fluid disorders	• Excess: diarrhea, facial edema, sweating. • Deficiency: dry mouth and throat, thirst, dry stool, concentrated urination, dry skin.	LI 11, 6, 4 LI 11, 4, 2	Lu 7, Ki 7, St 37, SI 3 Lu 10, Lu 7, Sp 6, Ki 6, UB 23
Heat Syndrome	• Yang Ming Channel Syndrome ("Four Greats") • Yang Ming Fu Syndrome (fever, hardness of stool, focal distention and abdominal pain). • Other febrile diseases.	LI 11, 2, 4 LI 11, 4, 2 LI 11, 4	Du 14, UB 40, St 44 St 37, St 44, St 25 SI 3, SJ 5, St 44, GB 43
Skin disorders	• Rashes, acne, eczema, boils, psoriasis.	LI 11, 4, 15	UB 40, Du 14, Lu 7, St 44, Ht 8
Large Intestine and Stomach disorders	• Abdominal pain, spasm, or distention, diarrhea, constipation, flatulence. • Epigastric pain, nausea, vomiting, belching.	LI 11, 4, 9, 8 LI 4, 11, 10	St 37, St 25, Sp 9, UB 25 Ren 12, St 36, Pc 6

The Clinical Applications (continued)

Category	Examples of Symptoms and Signs	Key points in order of importance.	Combinations with points from other channels.
Lung disorders	• Cough, asthma, sputum, chest pain.	LI 4, 11	Lu 7, Lu 5, Lu 6, Ren 17, UB 13
Qi and Blood Deficiency	• General lassitude, spontaneous sweating, dizziness, palpitations, low immunity.	LI 10, 4	Ren 6, St 36, UB 13, UB 17, UB 43

The Large Intestine Divergent Channel

Pathway

After separating from the Large Intestine Regular Channel at the hand, the Divergent Channel follows the Regular Channel up to the shoulder (LI 15 area). From this area, there are three branches.

The first branch goes posteriorly, connecting with the spinal column at the area of C7. The second goes anteriorly and distributes in the chest and breasts. The third goes to the supraclavicular fossa, where it enters the body cavity and connects with the lung and large intestine. It then travels upward, emerges at the supraclavicular fossa, passes through the throat, and converges with the Large Intestine Regular Channel, at the LI 18 area.

Separates at	Hand
Enters the body cavity at	Supraclavicular fossa
Connects with	Large intestine, lung, throat
Emerges from	Supraclavicular fossa
Converges with the Large Intestine Regular channel at	Throat (LI 18 area)

Clinical Applications

The Large Intestine Divergent Channel further reinforces the relationship between the large intestine and lungs. Clinically, points of the Large Intestine Channel can be used to treat the Lung disorders, and vice versa.

The Divergent Channel distributes in the chest and breast, extending the usage of the Large Intestine Channel to disorders of those areas. Examples include mastitis, fibrocystic breast disorders, myalgia, and chest pain. LI 10 and LI 11 are often used in combination with St 18, Ren 17, St 40, and Lv 3.

As LI 15 is the area from which the Divergent Channel divides into its three branches, this point can be used for disorders of the upper back, chest, lung, throat, and large intestine. It is often combined with LI 10, LI 11, LI 4, Lu 7, St 40, and Du 14.

LI 18 is the Converging Point. It can be used for such Large Intestine Channel disorders as arm pain, joint pain, tendinitis, and carpal tunnel syndrome. As the Converging point, it also has many applications for Lung Channel disorders. See also the Lung Divergent Channel for a full discussion.

The Large Intestine Tendinomuscular Channel

- Starts from: Index finger (LI 1).
- Ends at: Mandible.
- Qi accumulates at: Radial aspect of the wrist and elbow, shoulder, scapular region, spine, cheek, lateral side of the nose, corner of the head, and mandible.

Pathway

The Large Intestine Tendinomuscular Channel starts at the index finger, travels up the hand, and **knots**[1] at the wrist. From there, it goes up the forearm, **knots** at the lateral aspect of the elbow, continues up the upper arm, and **knots** at the shoulder (LI 15 area).

From the shoulder, a branch distributes over the scapula area, the Qi of which accumulates at the spine between the shoulder blades. The main portion of the Tendinomuscular Channel continues from the shoulder to the neck and cheek, where a branch separates and **knots** at the side of the nose. From the cheek, it continues upward on the lateral side of the face (anterior to the Small Intestine Tendinomuscular Channel), to the temporofrontal region. The three Yang Tendinomuscular Channels of Hand all knot at the temporofrontal area (around St 8). From there, it crosses over the top of the head, and ends at the mandible on the opposite side of the face.

Pathology

1. Spasm, pain, pulling sensation, and stiffness along the course of the Tendinomuscular Channel.
2. Impaired movement of the arm, shoulder stiffness, frozen shoulder.
3. Neck pain and stiffness, restricted rotation of the neck.

Clinical Applications

The primary applications of the Tendinomuscular Channel are pain, swelling, spasm, and hot and cold sensation along the channel distribution. The Tendinomuscular Channel can be used for arthritis, tendinitis, and carpal tunnel syndrome of the wrist, as well as arthritis and tendinitis of the elbow and shoulder. For example, tennis elbow can be effectively treated by applying Yang Ci[2] method to LI 10, LI 12, and GB 34 contralaterally.

The Tendinomuscular Channel has additional areas of distribution not covered by the Regular Channel. These include the scapular region, upper thoracic spine, and the distribution of m. trapezius. It is therefore useful for muscular disorders of these areas, from approximately C6 to T7. It is also used for cervical spondylosis, tightness, spasm, or trauma of the scapular region, and the area between the scapulae. It can further be used for tension and muscular spasm of m. trapezius, and the upper back. Points often used include LI 10, LI 11, LI 12, LI 4, in combination with Lu 7 and Lv 3 contralaterally.

While the Regular Channel circulates only around the mouth and nose, the Qi of the Tendinomuscular Channel accumulates at the cheek, side of the face, and mandible. This reinforces the theory that "the face is the field of Yang Ming," and supports the use of Large Intestine Channel points for disorders of the face and sense organs. Some examples are facial paralysis, TMJ syndrome, and trigeminal neuralgia.

Qi also accumulates at the temporofrontal region, where the three Yang Tendinomuscular Channels of the Hand meet, demonstrating that Large Intestine Channel points can be used for temporal as well as frontal headache. It is important to note that both the Regular and Tendinomuscular Channels end on the contralateral side of the body from which they began. This indicates that the selection of contralateral points would have a greater therapeutic effect, when treating disorders of the head and face.

---

[1] For an explanation of the significance of the *Jie (knots)* of the Tendinomuscular Channels, please refer to the Chapter of the Theory of the Twelve Channels, Section III. Characteristics of the Channel System, Subsection C. The Tendinomuscular Channels.

[2] See the Chapter of the Theory of the Twelve Channels, Section III. Characteristics of the Channel System, Subsection C. The Tendinomuscular Channels, acupuncture methods

Points often used for temporofrontal headache are LI 4 and LI 3, in combination with St 8, SJ 5 and GB 41.

The Luo Collateral of Large Intestine Channel

Luo point: LI 6
Distribution: It follows the main channel to LI 15, then to the angle of the mandible where it bifurcates. One branch enters the teeth, the other enters the ear, communicating with all the channels which go to the ear.
Connection: Shoulder, teeth, ear, Lung Channel
Notes: As LI 6 connects with the ear, the Large Intestine Channel system establishes its connection with all five sense organs.

Pathology
Excess: Toothache, gum disease, deafness, ear disorders.
Deficiency: Cold sensitivity or sensitive teeth, stifling sensation in the chest and diaphragm

Clinical Applications

Channel Disorders
1. Tooth disorders. Can be used for both excess and deficiency type including toothache, hot and cold sensitivity, gingivitis. Points used in combination with LI 6 are: St 44, LI 4, LI 7, Ki 6. St 6, St 7 SJ 17.
2. Ear disorders. Effective for ear disorders including deafness, ear ache, otitis media, tinnitus, and inflammation of the auricle. Points used in combination with LI 6 are: SJ 2, SJ 3, GB 42, GB 44, SJ 17, GB 2.
3. The Luo Collateral is applicable for other sense organ disorders such as redness of the eyes, sore throat, and epistaxis.

Organ Disorders
1. Disorders of the Body Fluids. As a Luo (Connecting) point, it is related to the Lung channel, the upper source of water. The Large Intestine Channel also dominates the disorders of body fluids. For these reasons, LI 6 can be effectively used for such disorders as general edema (especially upper portion of the body), retention of urine, and difficult urination. The combination points are: Lu 9, Lu 7, Ren 3, Ren 9, and St 40.[1]
2. Disorders of the chest and diaphragm. This point is useful for a variety of respiratory and epigastric disorders, such as stifling sensation and fullness, cough with sputum, food stagnation, bronchitis, gastritis and esophagus reflex. Points used in combination with LI 6 are: Lu 5, Ren 10, Ren 17, St 44 and St 40.

---

[1] As the Luo (Connecting) point of Large Intestine, this point has a relationship to the Lung channel, and thereby to the upper source of water.

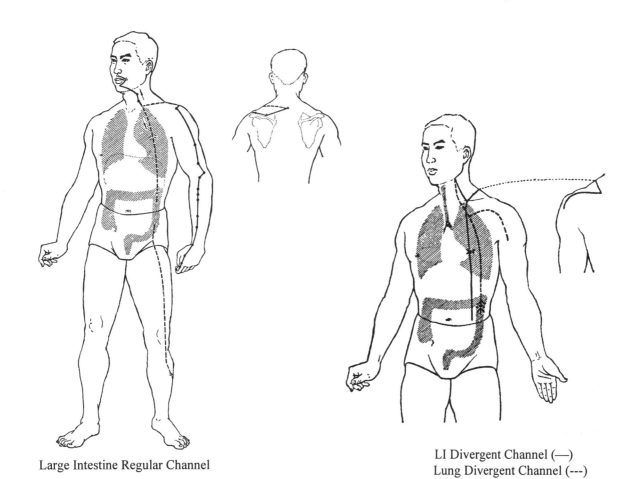

Large Intestine Regular Channel

LI Divergent Channel (—)
Lung Divergent Channel (---)

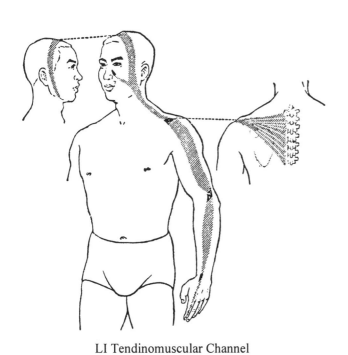

LI Tendinomuscular Channel

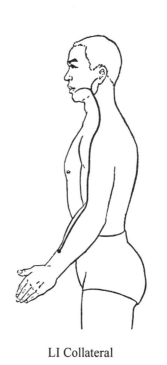

LI Collateral

The Large Intestine Channel of Hand-Yangming
手 陽 明 大 腸 經 系 統 分 布 圖

3. The Stomach Channel of Foot - Yang Ming
足 陽 明 胃 經

Key Points
- The Stomach Channel starts at the mid point of the infraorbital ridge (St 1).
- The channel ends at the medial aspect of the big toe (connects with the Spleen Channel at Sp 1).
- It distributes mainly on the face, neck, chest, abdomen, the lateroanterior aspect of the lower extremities, and the dorsum of foot.
- It connects with the stomach, spleen, and intestines.
- There are 45 points altogether.

The Pathway of the Stomach Regular Channel

External Pathway

The Stomach Regular Channel starts below the pupil at the infraorbital ridge (St 1). From there, it descends to the cheek, connects with the teeth in the upper gum, then goes to the philtrum (intersects Du 26). After intersecting the Du Channel, it curves around the upper lip to the mentolabial groove (intersects Ren 24). The channel then follows the mandible to the area anterior to the angle of the jaw. From there it changes direction, going upward (intersects GB 3). It reaches the temporofrontal region (St 8), which is 0.5 cun within the hairline, then travels medially to the Du channel (intersects Du 24). A branch from the cheek (St 5 area) goes down to the neck and supraclavicular fossa, then to the back (intersects Du 14).

From the supraclavicular fossa, the external portion of the channel descend the chest, passing through the nipple. It travels four cun lateral to the Ren channel while on the chest, then narrows to two cun lateral to it when it reaches the abdomen[1].

The external and internal branches diverge from each other at the supraclavicular fossa, and converge at the inguinal groove (St 30 area). The channel continues down the lateroanterior aspect of the thigh to the knee joint, then continues along the lateral aspect of the tibia to the dorsum of the foot, and ends at the lateral aspect of the 2nd toe. From St 36, a branch goes along m. tibialis and ends at the lateral aspect of the third toe. A second branch separates from St 42 (the highest point on the dorsum of the foot), then goes to the medial aspect of the big toe where it connects with the Spleen Channel (Sp 1).

Internal Pathway

The channel starts at the ala nasi (intersects LI 20) then goes along the sides of the nose to the bridge. Here, the left and right sides meet, before continuing to the medial aspect of the inner canthus (intersects UB 1). It then goes to the infraorbital ridge (St 1).

From the supraclavicular fossa, the internal pathway enters the body cavity, passes through the diaphragm, connects with the stomach (its pertaining organ), and connects with the spleen (intersects Ren 13, and 12 internally). A branch starts from the "lower orifice" of the stomach (duodenum), passes through the intestines, and emerges at the inguinal groove, where it rejoins the external pathway.

---

[1] Chapter 10, "Chapter of Channels" of the Nei Jing Ling Shu (Spiritual Axis) specifically mentions the Stomach Channel passing through the breast, nipple, the area lateral to the umbilicus, and the inguinal groove.

The Associated Organs and Points

Pertains to	Connects with	Associated With	Intersecting Points
Stomach	Spleen	Large intestine, small intestine, upper gum, heart (through the divergent channel), breast[1]	LI 20, UB 1, Ren 24, GB 3, GB 4, GB 6, Du 24, Du 26, Du 14, Ren 13, Ren 12, Sp 1

Physiology

The Stomach Channel has the following functions:

1. *Distribute Qi to the face and normalizes the function of the sense organs.* There is a saying, "The face is the field of the Yang Ming Channels." This means that both the Hand and Foot Yang Ming Channels nourish the face and sense organs, and regulate their functions. Disorders of the eyes, nose, gums, teeth, temporomandibular joint, and parotid gland, as well as acne and herpes lesions on the face, implicate a disorder of the Stomach Channel.

2. *Regulate the function of the digestive system.* This function should be understood to extend beyond the stomach organ itself to all the upper and lower digestive system. This includes the mouth, esophagus, stomach, spleen, pancreas, large and small intestines, gall bladder and liver, and the enzymatic secretions of digestion. These functions are primarily regulated by points on the lower leg, especially St 36, St 37, St 39, and St 40.

3. As a Yang Ming Channel, the Stomach Channel is considered a channel with "abundant Qi and Blood." In cases of Qi and Blood deficiency, points of the Stomach Channel are the source for tonification. St 36 and St 30[2], which are both "Sea of Nutrition" points, are commonly used. In cases of Qi and Blood excess, there may be mental disorders such as Dian Kuang syndrome (manic-depression), for which St 40 and St 37 are often used. When there is heat in the Qi and Blood, it may result in Yang Ming Channel syndrome, Yang Ming Fu syndrome, disorders of the skin, or Stomach Fire flaring up. In such cases, reducing method is often used on Stomach Channel points, such as St 44, St 37, and St 25.

4. *Nourish and strengthen the four extremities.* The Yang Ming Channel distributes Qi and the Blood to the four extremities. Therefore, its points can be used for *Bi syndrome*, or *Wei syndrome* (characterized by atrophy and flaccidity of the muscles).

Pathology

Channel Pathology from the Nei Jing

If the Stomach Channel is disordered, it results in *Gan Jue Syndrome*[3] *(Abnormality of the Shin).* Symptoms include aversion to cold with shivering, as if rain drops are hitting the body, sounds of distress (moaning), frequent yawning, dark complexion, and abdominal distention with borborygmus. In a serious case, the patient will dislike fire and the company other people, be frightened by "wood" sounds[4], have a feeling as if their heart is shaking (anxiety), and prefer to stay inside alone. As a further development, they may feel like going up to the roof and singing, taking off their clothing, and running or walking around outside.

---

[1] The Nei Jing says that the breast belongs to the Yang Ming (Stomach), and the nipple belongs to Jue Yin (Liver).

[2] There are four Seas: Sea of Qi, Sea of Blood, Sea of Nutrition and Sea of Marrow

[3] The distribution of the Stomach Channel covers the shin area. Gan Jue means the disorders of Stomach Channel. The points of this area are the most effective for treating these disorders.

[4] This is treated with St 37.

The Stomach Channel dominates the disorders of Blood, which includes illnesses caused by virulent and toxic febrile pathogens, malaria, and Dian Kuang Syndrome[1]. Other symptoms of the Stomach Channel disorders include profuse sweating, epistaxis, deviation of the mouth, herpes or blisters on the lips, swollen neck, throat disorders, abdominal edema, and swelling and pain of the knee joint. Also included are pain along the channel distribution on the chest, breast, inguinal groove, and thigh (especially around St 32), as well as on the lateral aspect of the tibia, the dorsum of the foot, and the toes.

If the Qi in the channel is deficient, there will be a cold sensation, or even shivering on the anterior of the body, including the chest and abdomen. There will also be indigestion or retention of food in the stomach, which causes fullness and distention. This is due to Yang deficient cold. If the Qi in the channel is in excess, there will be a sensation of heat on the front of the body, and excess heat in stomach which causes the patient to become easily hungry. There may also be yellow urination.

Summary of Channel Pathology

Dominates Disorders of	Blood
Channel Disorders	• <u>Heat Syndrome (Yang Ming Channel Syndrome)</u>: "Four Greats": (profuse sweating, extreme thirst, high fever, surging pulse), shivering (as in malaria), a red face, coma, delirium, yellow urination. • <u>Head, Face and Sense Organs</u>: painful eyes, dry nose or epistaxis, lip and mouth ulcers including herpes, painful throat, swollen neck, and deviation of the mouth, toothache, and frontal headache. • <u>Channel Obstruction</u>: pain, muscle spasm, redness, swelling or coldness on the front of the thigh and leg, and on the foot. • <u>Breast Disorders</u>: redness, pain and swelling of the breast, fibrocystic breast disorder.
Organ Disorders	• <u>Yang Ming Fu Syndrome</u>: fever, constipation with hard stools, focal distention and fullness of the abdomen, yellow urination. • <u>Stomach Disorders</u>: frequent hunger and feeling of emptiness in the stomach (the stomach is quickly emptied due to a high metabolic rate), indigestion, distention and pain of the epigastrium, nausea and vomiting. • <u>Intestinal Disorders</u>: abdominal distention, fullness and pain, diarrhea, constipation, borborygmus, abdominal edema (including liver cirrhosis, blockage of the portal vein). • <u>Dian/Kuang Syndrome</u>: (manic-depression), abnormal mental function, violent behavior, abnormal yawning and moaning.

The Clinical Applications

The Stomach Channel is mainly applied to treat digestive disorders, including such biomedically defined disorders as gastritis, peptic ulcer, duodenal ulcer, nervous stomach, hiatal hernia, pancreatitis, hepatitis, cholecystitis, and cholelithiasis. It can also be used for disorders of the blood, which mainly include febrile diseases and mental disorders. The Stomach Channel is also effective for disorders of the head and face, as well as those disorders which occur along the channel's distribution.

---

[1] Dian Kuang syndrome expressed itself as violent, out of control behavior.

The Clinical Applications (continued)

Category	Examples of Symptoms and Signs	Key points in order of importance.	Combinations with points from other channels.
Digestive Disorders	• Excess: epigastric pain, nausea, vomiting, belching, easily hungry, nervous eating, constipation, diarrhea, borborygmus, abdominal fullness and distention. Burning sensation in the stomach with sour regurgitation, and Yang Ming Fu Syndrome	St 44, 34, 25, 40, 37	Ren 10, Ren 13, Pc 6, Sp 4, UB 44, Sp 2, Lv 2
	• Deficiency: epigastric pain, poor appetite, indigestion, abdominal distention, diarrhea, constipation, cold sensation in the stomach.	St 36, 37, 39, 30, 21	Ren 12, Sp 3, Lv 13, UB 20, UB 21, Pc 6, Sp 6
Head, Face and Sense Organ Disorders	• Head: Yang Ming headache	St 43, 44, 8	LI 4, LI 3
	• Eye: pain, redness of the eyes	St 1, 2, 44	LI 3, LI 4, Lv 2, GB 37, GB 20
	• Nose: rhinitis, sinusitis, epistaxis, nose obstruction.	St 2, 3, 37, 41	UB 57, LI 4, LI 11, Lu 7, Sp 3, GB 41
	• Throat: swollen throat, thyroid disorders	St 44, 40, 9, 10	LI 2, LI 4, SJ 10, SJ 13, LI 18, SI 2, Ki 6
	• Toothache and gum disorders	St 5, 6, 7, 44, 43	LI 4, LI 7, Ki 6, SJ 17
	• Facial paralysis, TMJ syndrome, trigeminal neuralgia	St 4, 6, 7, 36, 37	LI 4, LI 10, SJ 17
	• Herpes of the lips, ulceration of the mouth	St 4, 36, 44	Ren 24, LI 4, Sp 6, Sp 2
Qi and Blood Deficiency	• General lassitude, sallow complexion, shortness of breath, spontaneous sweating, palpitations, scanty menstruation	St 36, 30, 37, 39, 42	LI 10, Ren 6, UB 17, UB 20, UB 21
Heat Syndromes	• Yang Ming Channel or Qi Level syndrome: high fever (or shivering), profuse sweating, great thirst, surging pulse, or with cough, yellow sputum, and chest pain.	St 44, 45, 40	LI 11, Du 14
	• Excessive Stomach Fire: acute stomach pain, burning sensation, vomiting, bleeding gums.	St 44, 40, 41, 34	Lu 6, Lu 5, Pc 5, SJ 5
Mental Disorders (Dian/Kuang Syndrome)	• Violent behavior	St 40, 45	Select from the 13 Ghost Points[1]
	• Withdrawn behavior	St 40, 25, 8, 37	Select from the 13 Ghost Points
Breast Disorders	• Swelling, pain, redness, fibrocystic disorder of breast	St 40, 44, 36, 37, 39, 18	LI 11, SI 1, Ren 17, GB 21

---

[1] Sun Si Miao in the book *Qian Jin Yao Fang* lists Du 26, Lu 11, Sp 1, Pc 7, UB 62, Du 16, St 6, Ren 24, Pc 8, Du 23, Ren 1, LI 11, Jin Jin/Yu Ye (extra points) as the thirteen Ghost Points. A later generation added two points: Pc 5, SI 3.

The Clinical Applications (continued)

Category	Examples of Symptoms and Signs	Key points in order of importance.	Combinations with points from other channels.
Channel Disorders	• Pain, muscle spasms, hot and cold sensations along the channel distribution.	St 43, 36, 37, 39, 32, 31, 40	LI 15, LI 11, LI 4, SJ 5, GB 34, Lv 3, UB 65
	• Wei Syndrome: weakness and atrophy of the muscles of the whole body.	St 36, 32, 41	LI 10, LI 4, LI 15, Sp 21, Lv 8, Du 4, Du 3, UB 21, UB 20

The Stomach Divergent Channel

Pathway

After separating from the Regular Channel on the anterior aspect of the thigh, the Stomach Divergent Channel goes to the inguinal groove (St 30 area). From this area, it enters the body cavity and connects with the stomach and spleen, then goes upward to connect with the heart. From there it travels along the sides of the esophagus and throat, emerges at the mouth, continues upward along the sides of the nose, and finally connects with the eye system near the inner canthus (UB 1 area). Here, it converges with the Stomach Regular Channel.

Summary

Separates from	Thigh
Enters the body cavity at	Inguinal groove (St 30 area)
Connects with	Stomach, spleen, heart, esophagus, throat, mouth, eye system
Emerges from	Mouth
Converges with Stomach Regular channel at	Inner canthus (UB 1 area)

Clinical Applications

The Stomach Divergent Channel reinforces the relationship between the Stomach and Spleen, supporting the selection of Stomach Channel points for treating disorders of the Spleen, and vice versa. It connects with the heart, providing the theoretical basis for selecting Stomach Channel points for the treatment of heart disorders. For instance, indigestion or hiatal hernia may cause insomnia[1], and disorders of the Mind (heart) may cause poor appetite and epigastric pain. In either case, Stomach points, such as St 36 and St 40, are used for treatment, in combination with Pc 6, Ht 7, and Ren 10.

The Stomach Divergent Channel further distributes Qi to the face and sense organs. That is why Stomach points can often be effective in treating sinusitis, Yang Ming headache due to stomach disorders, and food allergies. Points often used are St 43, St 44, St 36, and St 37.

The Divergent Channel reinforces the connection between the Stomach Channel and the eye system, demonstrating the strong Qi connection between St 30 and the eyes. Flushing of the face, and redness, swelling, and pain of the eyes, are often due to excessive Qi and Blood rushing to the eyes. Reducing method or pricking technique on St 30, treats these conditions by directing heat downward.

---

[1] This is called Disturbed sleep due to Disharmony of the Stomach and Heart.

The Stomach Tendinomuscular Channel

- Starts from: 2nd, 3rd, and 4th toes
- Ends at: In front of the ear
- Qi accumulates at: St 41, the lateral aspect of the knee joint, hip, spine, lateral patella, front
  of the thigh, external genitalia, supraclavicular fossa, nose, lower lid, and ear.

Pathway

The Stomach Tendinomuscular Channel starts from the 2nd, 3rd and 4th toes, travels to dorsum of foot, and **knots** around St 41. It then goes upward, distributing along the fibula, and **knots** on the lateral aspect of the knee joint. It continues upward on the lateral side of the leg (approximating the Gall Bladder Regular Channel line), and **knots** at the hip joint. From there, it passes through the hypochondriac region, and to the back, where it connects with the spinal column.

A branch separates on the lower leg, follows m. tibialis to the lateral patella, where it **knots** and **converges** with the Gall Bladder Tendinomuscular Channel. It also re-connects with the main portion of Stomach Tendinomuscular Channel in this area. The Stomach Tendinomuscular Channel continues up the thigh along m. quadriceps, and **knots** around St 31. It then goes transversely to the external genitalia, where it **converges** with several other tendinomuscular channels. Continuing upward, it distributes in the abdomen, passes through the chest, and **knots** at the supraclavicular fossa. From there, it extends to the neck, face, sides of the mouth, and **knots** beside the nose. From the nose it connects with the lower eyelid where it **converges** with the Urinary Bladder Tendinomuscular Channel. Together, these two tendinomuscular channels form a network connecting the upper and lower lids. A branch separates from the jaw, goes across the cheek, and **knots** in front of the ear.

Pathology

1. Stiffness and pulling of the toes.
2. Leg muscle spasms, including the gastrocnemius.
3. Throbbing, hardness, and stiffness of the dorsum of the foot (St 41 area).
4. Spasm of m. quadriceps (St 32 and St 31 area).
5. Swelling and distention of the inguinal groove area.
6. Hernia.
7. Abdominal muscle spasms, pain and spasms of the supraclavicular fossa and face.
8. Sudden deviation of the mouth[1].
9. Spasm or drooping of the eyelids which are then unable to open.

Clinical Applications

The main application of the Stomach Tendinomuscular Channel is treating pain, muscle spasm, hot and cold sensations, numbness, and paralysis along the channel distribution. The dorsum of the foot and all four toes are connected by the Stomach Tendinomuscular Channel, indicating that Stomach points are of primary importance for treating foot disorders.

The Stomach Regular and Divergent Channels are distributed on the front of the trunk and the lower extremities. The Tendinomuscular Channel extends the distribution to the lateral side of the trunk and lower extremities, including the fibula, lateral side of the knee, thigh, hip, hypochondriac region, and back. These areas approximate the distribution of the Gall Bladder Channel. Disorders such as spasm and pain of the hypochondriac region and back, sciatica, and hip joint pain can be treated by St 36 and St 40.

The Stomach Regular Channel passes through the inguinal groove, but the Tendinomuscular Channel extends to the external genitalia. This indicates that Stomach Channel points are applicable to urogenital disorders such as cystitis, vaginitis, hernia, orchitis, and herpes. Points often used include St 30, St 39, St 40, and St 44, in combination with Lv 5, Sp 9, and Ren 1.

---

[1] If there is heat in the Tendinomuscular Channel, there will be paralysis, loss of muscle tone, inability to open the eye, and deviation of the mouth. If there is cold, it causes a spasm which deviates the mouth to the opposite side.

Because of the Tendinomuscular Channel's connection with the eyelids, Stomach points can be used for puffiness, blepharoptosis (drooping of the eyelids), and inability to close the eyelids due to facial paralysis. St 1, 36, and 43 are often applied.

The Yang Ming Channels have a strong influence on the entire face and the sense organs. The Stomach Regular and Divergent Channels connect with the mouth, nose, and eyes. The Tendinomuscular Channel extends the connection to the ears, completing the theory (initially presented in the chapter on the Large Intestine Channel) that the Yang Ming Channels connect with all the sense organs. This supports the selection of Stomach points for disorders of the face and sense organs, including disorders of the ear, such as tinnitus, otitis media, and deafness. St 36, St 44, St 40, and St 43 are commonly used.

The Luo Collateral of Stomach Channel

Luo point: St 40

Distribution: After separating from the Stomach Regular Channel at St 40, the Luo Collateral makes a network connecting with the Spleen Channel. It then follows the Stomach Regular Channel to the supraclavicular fossa, where it bifurcates. One branch goes to the throat. The other goes to the head and nape, where it communicates with all Yang Qi. It then enters the brain.

Connection: Throat, nape, brain, Spleen Channel.

Pathology

Excess: Mental disorders, including Dian and Kuang syndrome. Schizophrenia, manic-depression, insanity, and epilepsy are a few examples.

Deficiency: Atrophy, weakness, and flaccidity of the muscles of the leg and feet, especially in the shin area.

Rebellious Qi: Obstruction of throat, swelling and painful throat, and sudden hoarseness (sudden aphasia).

Clinical Applications

Channel Disorders

1. <u>Wei and Bi Syndrome</u>. Stomach Luo Collateral is important for treating Wei and Bi syndromes of the lower extremities, manifesting with such symptoms as muscular atrophy, and pain and swelling of the lower extremities and feet. Points used in combination with St 40 are St 36, 32, GB 31, GB 39.
2. <u>Throat Disorders</u>. Because of its connection to the throat the Luo Collateral is applied to such throat disorders as swelling and pain of the throat, sudden hoarseness, Plum Pit Qi, and thyroid disorders. Points used in combination with St 40 are LI 1, 3, 4, Lu 10, 7, Ht 5, and Ki 6.

Organ Disorders

1. <u>Stomach and Spleen Disorders</u>. The Luo Collateral is applied to the disorders of both Spleen and Stomach, such as epigastric pain, loose stools, poor appetite, and abdominal distention. St 40 is an important point for both substantial and non-substantial phlegm.
2. <u>Mental Disorders</u>. As the Stomach Lou Connecting point is directly related to the brain, it is very effective for treating mental disorders, such as phlegm misting the heart manifesting in manic-depression, schizophrenia, and epilepsy. St 40, which is itself a Ghost Point, is often combined with a selection of several other Ghost Points, St 45, Sp 1, Pc 5, Du 20, and Du 16 for example.
3. <u>Chest and Lung Disorders</u>. Substantial phlegm with cough and sputum, asthma, bronchitis, pneumonia and dyspnea, can be treated with St 40 in combination with Lu 5, Lu 7, LI 4, Ki 6, Ren 12, and St 41.

4. Phlegm Accumulation Disorders. Swollen glands, nodules, masses, and tumors, which result from accumulation of phlegm, can also be treated by St 40 in combination with Sp 3, SJ 3, SJ 17, UB 21, and UB 22.

The Stomach Great Luo Collateral

Luo point: Xu Li. Located on the left side of the chest where the heart beat can be seen. Approximately St 18[1].

Distribution: From Xu Li, the Stomach Great Luo Collateral goes down to the stomach, then up to penetrate the diaphragm, and connects with the lung. Its distribution is mainly on the left side of the breast where the heart beat can be palpated.

Connection: Heart, stomach, diaphragm, and lung.

Pathology

Excess: Rapid breathing, irregular breathing, dyspnea.

Deficiency: Compression and suffocating sensation in the chest as in asthmatic breathing, cough, angina pectoris and heart attack..

Clinical Applications

This point is used for local respiratory and heart disorders, such as asthma, dyspnea, emphysema, and bradycardia. It can also be applied for hysteria or anxiety attacks, with gasping for breath. While practicing in the China, the author observed the effective use of this point, in combination with others, for the emergency treatment of angina pectoris and heart attack.

---

[1] This point is contraindicated for moxibustion because it is over the heart. Shallow needle insertion is required.

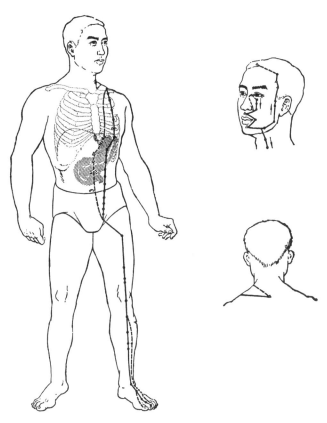

Stomach Regular Channel

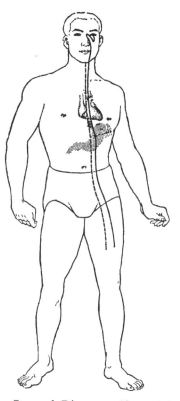

Stomach Divergent Channel (—)
Spleen Divergent Channel (---)

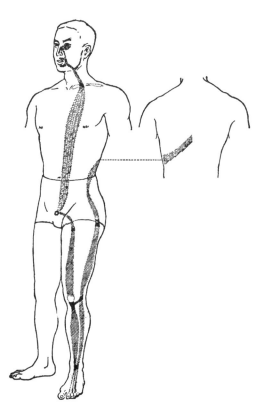

Stomach Tendinomuscular Channel

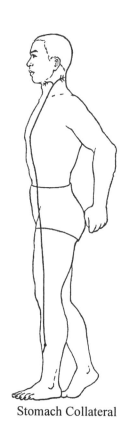

Stomach Collateral

The Stomach Channel of Foot-Yangming
足 陽 明 胃 經 系 統 分 布 圖

4. The Spleen Channel of Foot - Tai Yin

足 太 陰 脾 經

Key Points

- The Spleen Channel starts on the medial aspect of the big toe (Sp 1).
- The channel ends at the side of the chest (Sp 21) externally, and the heart internally.
- It distributes mainly on the medioanterior aspect of the lower extremities, abdomen, chest, and to the tongue.
- It connects with the spleen, stomach, and the heart.
- There are 21 points altogether.

The Pathway of the Spleen Regular Channel

External Pathway

The Spleen Regular Channel starts from the big toe (Sp 1), goes along the medial aspect of the foot, in front of the medial malleolus, then to the medial aspect of the lower leg. The rule of channel distribution states that on the extremities, the Jue Yin Channel should travel between the Tai Yin and the Shao Yin Channels, i.e., the Liver Channel should travel between the Spleen and Kidney Channels. The lower leg is an exception to this rule. Starting from the foot, and until it reaches the level of eight cun above the medial malleolus, the Liver channel travels anteriorly, rather than posteriorly to the Spleen Channel. Above this level the channels go back to their regular pattern.

From the lower leg, the channel continues to the medial aspect of the thigh, then passes through the inguinal groove. As it goes up the abdomen, it holds to a line four cun lateral to the midline of the abdomen (intersects Ren 3, Ren 4, and Ren 10). When it reaches the chest, its distance from the midline increases to six cun lateral (intersects GB 24, Lv 14, and Lu 1). The external pathway ends at the side of the chest (Sp 21).

Internal Pathway

The channel enters the body cavity at the inguinal groove (Sp 12 area), then connects with its pertaining organ, the spleen, and connects with the stomach. From the stomach, it passes through the diaphragm, along the sides the esophagus, then further upward to connect with the root of the tongue. It ends by dispersing on the tongue's lower surface. A branch from the stomach passes through the diaphragm and flows into the heart, where it connects with the Heart Channel.

The Associated Organs and Points

Pertains to	Connects with	Associated With	Intersecting Points
Spleen	Stomach	Heart, tongue, esophagus, diaphragm	Ren 3, Ren 4, Ren 10, GB 24, Lv 14, Lu 1

Physiology

The functions of the Spleen Channel are similar to those of the Spleen in Zang Fu theory. They include the digestive functions of the stomach, small intestine, pancreas, certain functions of liver and gall bladder, and the digestive enzymes. The Spleen Channel has the following functions:

1. *Promote and regulate the digestion and absorption of food and drink.* Symptoms such as poor appetite, abdominal distention, and diarrhea are indicative of a Spleen Channel disorder.
2. *Regulate the transportation of body fluids and prevent the formation of dampness in the Middle Jiao.* Symptoms such as heavy sensation of the head, body, and extremities, edema, excessive salivation, and diarrhea are indications of dampness in the interior, which can be treated by Spleen Channel points.
3. *Tonify Qi and Blood.* The Ying (Nutritive Qi) is produced by the Spleen, and distributed through its channel to the whole body. Qi and Blood deficiency, with symptoms such as general lassitude, fatigue, insomnia, and profuse menstrual flow, can be treated with points such as Sp 3, Sp 4, and Sp 6.
4. *Raise and stabilize the Qi.* The Spleen Channel sends the Clear Qi upward to nourish the head and the face. It also strengthens the smooth muscles of the internal organs and ligaments which hold the organs in their proper place. Symptoms such as dizziness, light-headedness, difficulty concentrating, and prolapse of the organs, indicate a disorder of Spleen Channel.
5. *Nourish the muscles and extremities.* The Spleen and Stomach are the source of Qi and Blood. They dominate the muscles and the four extremities. This is why Spleen and Stomach points can be used for *Wei syndrome*, which is characterized by atrophy and flaccidity of the muscles.

Pathology

Channel Pathology from the Nei Jing

The Spleen Channel dominates the disorders of the Spleen. If the Spleen is disordered, there will be epigastric pain, abdominal distention relieved by passing gas, vomiting after eating, belching easily, poor appetite, diarrhea or loose stools, water retention, jaundice, spasm and pain below the heart (epigastric pain), anxiety, restlessness, difficulty sleeping, stiffness and pain of the tongue, heavy sensation of the body, and difficulty standing. There will also be pain, swelling, and coldness along the medial thigh and knee, and impaired movement of the big toe.

Summary of Channel Pathology

Dominates Disorders Of	Spleen
Channel Disorder	• Dampness in the Channels: heavy sensation of the head and body, facial puffiness, swelling of the legs, feet, and joints • Tongue Disorders: loss of capability to roll or extend the tongue, stiffness of the tongue, impaired speech. • Channel Obstruction: pain, coldness, or heat sensation along the medial thigh, knee, leg, foot and toe, pain in the cheek and mandible. • Wei Syndrome: flaccidity or atrophy of the muscles, especially of the extremities.
Organ Disorder	• Stomach and Spleen Disorders: epigastric pain, loose stools, diarrhea, borborygmus, vomiting, nausea, abdominal fullness and distention, reduced appetite, jaundice, general lassitude and listlessness, and abdominal Qi masses. • Water retention and dampness: edema, excessive phlegm fluid, difficult urination, excessive leukorrhea.

Differentiation of Stomach and Spleen Pathology

The Stomach often shows symptoms of excess, such as frequent hunger and excessive appetite, while the Spleen commonly demonstrates symptoms of deficiency and chronic digestive disorders, such as poor or reduced appetite. Nausea and vomiting more likely will implicate a Stomach disorder, while Spleen disorders are more likely to result in loose stools and abdominal distention.

Nausea, vomiting, and belching may be related to either the Stomach or Spleen. If the Stomach is involved, the symptoms usually occur directly after eating. If Spleen is involved, the symptoms are generally more chronic and usually occur a long time after eating.

The Clinical Applications

The Spleen Channel is mainly used for the disorders of the digestive system and urogenital system.

Category	Examples of Symptoms and Signs	Key points in order of importance.	Combinations with points from other channels.
Digestive Disorders	Deficiency: poor appetite, loose stools, abdominal distention, borborygmus, constipation.	Sp 3, 6, 4, 15	UB 20, St 36, Pc 6
	Excess: epigastric and abdominal distention and pain, nausea, vomiting, diarrhea.	Sp 9, 2, 4	St 40, Pc 6, Pc 5, St 37
Disorders Caused by Dampness	Edema, heavy sensation of the head, body and extremities, sleepiness after eating, excessive salivation, diarrhea, eczema, accumulation of phlegm fluid, abnormal discharge (e.g., nasal, vaginal, ear, skin)	Sp 3, 9, 6, 7, 5, 21	St 40, SJ 6, Lu 7, Ren 9, UB 22
	Hypercholesterolemia, obesity, atherosclerosis, masses and nodules.	Sp 9, 6, 3	St 40, UB 20, SJ 9, Pc 6, UB 22
Deficiency of Qi and Blood	Qi and Blood Deficiency: lassitude, fatigue, dizziness, headache, insomnia, sallow complexion, bruising or bleeding easily, coagulation disorders	Sp 3, 4, 6, 10, 21	St 36, UB 20, Ren 12, UB 17, Ren 6
	Sinking of Qi: prolapsed stomach, kidney, uterus, rectum, hernia, dizziness, vertigo, lightheadedness.	Sp 3, 6	St 36, Du 20, UB 20
Urogenital Disorders	Irregular menstruation, menorrhagia, metrorrhagia, amenorrhea, infertility, dysmenorrhea, leukorrhea, genital herpes or eczema, unsmooth urination, retention of urine.	Sp 1, 8, 3, 4, 6, 10	Lv 3, Lv 5, Lv 8, Ren 4, Ren 3, UB 20, St 36, Ki 6
Emotional Disorders	Constant worrying, low spirits, difficulty concentrating, poor memory, depression, palpitations.	Sp 6, 10, 4	St 40, Ht 7, Pc 6, Du 20, SJ 3, Ki 4, UB 20

The Clinical Applications (continued)

Channel Disorders	<u>Channel Obstruction</u>: pain, heaviness, swelling, cold sensation along the channel distribution.	Sp 3, 5, 9	St 40, GB 34, St 36, Lv 3
	<u>Wei Syndrome</u>: atrophy and flaccidity of the muscles, especially on the lower extremities.	Sp 3, 6, 9, 21	St 36, GB 31, GB 39, St 40

The Spleen Divergent Channel

Pathway

After separating from the Spleen Regular Channel on the thigh, the Spleen Divergent Channel joins the Stomach Divergent Channel at the inguinal groove. It then flows along with it up to, and connects with, the throat, then further upward to penetrate and connect with the tongue.

Summary

Separates at	Thigh
Enters the abdomen at	Inguinal groove (Sp 12, St 30 area)
Connects with	Stomach, spleen, heart, esophagus, throat, mouth and tongue.
Emerges from	Throat
Converges with Stomach Regular Channel at	Mouth

Clinical Applications

The Spleen Divergent Channel emphasizes the relationship between the Spleen and the Stomach, supporting the selection of Spleen points for disorders of the Stomach, and vice versa. Clinically, Spleen points can be used for disorders of the whole digestive system.

The Divergent Channel reinforces the connection between the spleen and the heart. Deficiency of Qi and Blood, and mental disorders, can be treated with Spleen points, such as Sp 3 and Sp 4, in combination with Pc 6 and Ht 7.

St 30 is the area where the Spleen and Stomach Divergent Channels converge before entering the body cavity. It is also a Sea of Nutrition point. This makes it very important for treating digestive disorders, such as distention, pain, and spasm of the abdomen, flatulence, diarrhea, borborygmus, hematemesis, and tarry stools.

The Spleen Divergent Channel emphasizes the connection between the Spleen Channel and the throat. Sp 3, in combination with St 40 and Pc 5, is effective for damp phlegm accumulating in the throat, causing chronic throat and thyroid disorders.

The Spleen Divergent Channel makes an additional connection with the tongue and mouth. This supports the choice of Sp 3, Sp 2, and Sp 6 for the treatment of tongue and mouth disorders. Some examples include sores or ulcers of the mouth and tongue, stiffness of the tongue, and unclear speech due to damp phlegm accumulating at the tongue.

The Spleen Tendinomuscular Channel

- Starts from: The medial side of the big toe.
- Ends at: The spinal column.

- Qi accumulates at: Medial malleolus, medial aspect of the knees, inguinal groove, umbilicus, ribs, chest, and spine.

Pathway
From the medial aspect of the big toe, the Spleen Tendinomuscular Channel goes upward to the medial malleolus **(knots),** continues up and **knots** on the medial aspect of the knee. It then traverses the medial aspect of the thigh and **knots** at the inguinal groove, where it joins the external genitalia. It then goes upward to connect with the umbilicus **(knots),** enters internally, knots at the ribs, and disperses in the chest. A branch from the ribs arches upward and then down, connecting with the spine.

Pathology
1. Pulling sensation and stiffness of the big toe.
2. Pain of the medial malleolus.
3. Spasm and pain on the medial aspect of the leg and knee.
4. Spasm and pain on the medial aspect of the thigh (m. adductor longus), referring to the inguinal groove.
5. Spasm, pulling pain, or cold sensation of the external genitalia.
6. Pain of the umbilicus that refers to the hypochondriac region.
7. Pulling pain of the intercostal regions that refers to the spinal column.

Clinical Applications
The primary applications of the Spleen Tendinomuscular Channel include treating pain, muscle spasms, hot and cold sensations, numbness, and paralysis along the channel distribution, especially on the medial aspect of the lower extremities.

The Tendinomuscular Channel extends a connection to the external genitalia. Therefore, it can be used to treat pulling pain, spasm, and abnormal discharge of that area. Disorders such as swelling of the scrotum, epididymitis, prostatitis, pain, swelling or nodules of the labia, hernia, herpes, and excess vaginal discharge can be treated. For these conditions, Sp 4, Sp 5, Sp 6 and Sp 9 are often used in combination with Lv 5, GB 41 and SJ 5.

The Tendinomuscular Channel also connects with the umbilicus. This emphasizes the Spleen Channel's application for treating cold damp accumulation, resulting in abdominal pain, spasm, coldness, or sweating of the umbilicus. Sp 3 and Ren 8 are often treated with moxibustion.

Because of this channel's connection with the spine, digestive disorders can be reflected on the back, and pain and spasm of the back may refer to the abdomen. Spleen points such as Sp 3, Sp 4, and Sp 7 can be used in combination with UB 20 and UB 21 in either case.

The Luo Collateral of Spleen Channel

Luo point:	Sp 4
Distribution:	After separating from the Spleen Regular Channel, the Luo Collateral immediately connects with the Stomach Channel, then it follows the Spleen Regular Channel, enters the abdominal cavity, and connects with the intestines and stomach.
Connection:	Stomach, intestines, Stomach Channel

Pathology
Excess:	Colic pain of the stomach and intestines
Deficiency:	*Gu Zhang* (Drum Abdominal Distention) such as ascites, childhood nutritional impairment, flatulence, abdominal fullness, and distention.
Rebellious Qi:	Acute vomiting, diarrhea, severe abdominal pain, and dehydration, such as in an acute attack of cholera.

Clinical Applications

The area influenced by Sp 4 is the abdomen, especially below the umbilicus. Sp4 can be used for digestive and urogenital disorders.

Organ Disorders

1. Digestive Disorders. Sp 4 is especially effective for abdominal pain and distention, spastic colon, ulcerative colitis, enteritis, irritable bowel syndrome, diverticulitis and dysentery including cases where accompanied by vomiting, nausea, and diarrhea. Points used in combination with Sp 4 are: Pc 6, St 37, St 25, LI 4, and LI 11. It also works well in treating flatulence, ascites, childhood nutritional impairment (which causes protrusion of the abdomen), or a large, obese abdomen. For these disorders, Sp 4 is used in combination with Pc 6, LI 11, 10, St 36, and Sp 15.
2. Urogenital Disorders. Sp 4 is useful for pain and distention of the lower abdomen due to dysmenorrhea, PMS, uroschesis, and cystitis in combination with Sp 8, Pc 6, Lv 5, Ren 3 and Shiqizhuixia.

Channel Disorders

Sp 4 is potent in treating disorders of the foot, such as plantar fascitis, heel spurs, hot sensation in the sole of the foot, arthritis, and bunions. Points used in combination with Sp 4 are: Sp 3, Lv 3, UB 62, Ki 4 and Ki 2.

The Spleen Great Luo Collateral

Luo point:	Sp 21.
Distribution:	After separating from the Regular Channel at Sp 21, six cun below the axillary fossa, the Spleen Great Luo Collateral then distributes to, and spreads into the chest and hypochondriac region.
Connection:	None.

Pathology

Excess:	Whole body pain, multiple site arthritis, Bi syndrome.
Deficiency:	Muscular atrophy and flaccidity, weakness of the joints , weakness of the whole body.

Clinical Applications

The function of the Fourteen Luo Collaterals is to distribute Qi and Blood through a network which covers the front and back of the body and the extremities. The Great Luo Collateral of the Spleen Channel extends this network to the lateral aspects of the trunk. Sp 21 serves as a center for this distribution, nourishing, and balancing the whole body through the small, fine, and minute collaterals.

The Spleen Great Luo Collateral can be used for the following conditions:

1. Pain of the whole body, such as multiple site arthritis, Bi Syndrome, fibromyalgia, multiple sclerosis, Lupus, and Crone's disease. Points used in combination with Sp 21 are: Du 14, UB 11, UB 65, SI 3 and Lv 8. It should be noted that Sp 21 is contraindicated in initial stages of flu-related body aches and joint pain because it is too Yin, and its use may pull the pathogen inward.
2. Weakness of the body, such as muscular atrophy or flaccidity and weakness of the joints, deficient syndromes such as deficiency of Qi, Blood, Yin and Yang of the organs, post-surgical and post-partum weakness, and chronic fatigue syndrome. Points used in combination with Sp 21 are: St 36, Ren 4, Ren 6, UB 17, UB 43, and UB23.

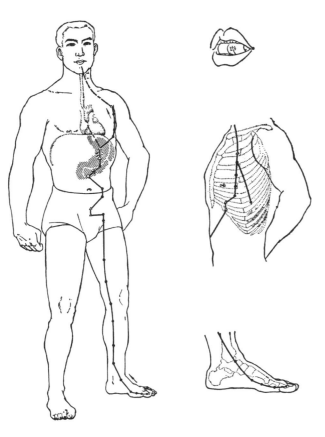

Spleen Regular Channel

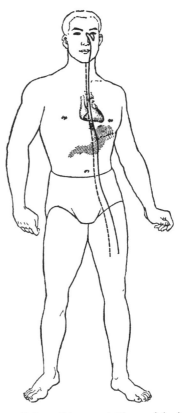

Spleen Divergent Channel (---)
Stomach Divergent Channel (——)

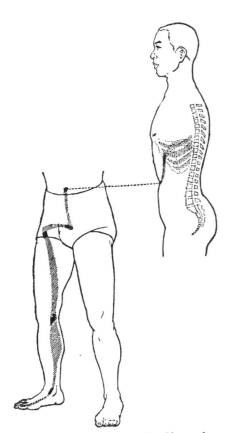

Spleen Tendinomuscular Channel

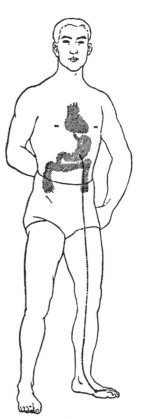

Spleen Collateral

The Spleen Channel of Foot-Taiyin

足太陰脾經系統分布圖

5. The Heart Channel of Hand - Shao Yin

手 少 陰 心 經

Key Points

- The Heart Channel starts in the heart.
- The channel ends at the radial aspect of the small finger (Ht 9), where it connects with the Small Intestine Channel.
- It distributes mainly on the medioposterior aspect of the arm and axillary fossa.
- It connects with the heart and small intestine.
- There are 9 points altogether.

The Pathway of the Heart Regular Channel

Internal Pathway

The internal pathway begins at the heart, comes down through the diaphragm and connects with the small intestine at the Ren 4 area. A branch separates from the Heart system[1], goes upward along the sides of the esophagus to the face, and connects with the eye system[2]. Another branch goes to, and through the Lungs from the Heart system, then emerges at the axillary fossa.

External Pathway

From the axillary fossa, the external pathway follows the medioposterior aspect of the upper arm, elbow and forearm. It then passes through the palm to the radial side of the small finger, where it connects with the Small Intestine Channel (SI 1).

The Associated Organs and Points

Pertains to	Connects with	Associated With	Intersecting Points
Heart	Small intestine	Lung, esophagus, eye system	None

Physiology

The Heart Channel has the following functions:

1. *Circulate the Qi and Blood, nourish the heart, lungs, and eyes.* Symptoms such as cardiac pain, insomnia, palpitations, restlessness, stifling sensation in the chest, and change of facial complexion may implicate a disorder of the Heart Channel.
2. *Regulate the nervous system, calm the mind, and stabilize the emotions.* Symptoms such as mental or emotional disorders, hysteria, anxiety, nervousness, and laughing or crying without apparent reason, may implicate a disorder of the Heart Channel. Because the Heart perceives all sensations, pain and itching regardless of etiology, can be treated with Heart points.
3. *Regulate heat in the body.* As a Fire element channel, Heart has a regulating function on heat of the body. Symptoms such as thirst and dry throat, hot sensation of the body, hot palms, boils, carbuncles, and redness of the eyes, may be treated by Heart points.

---

[1] The Heart system includes the pericardium, arteries, nerves and tissues surrounding the heart.

[2] The Eye system includes the tissues, nerves and vessels around and behind the eyes which directly relate to the brain.

4. *Distribute Qi and Blood to the areas covered by the Heart Channel.* This includes the medioposterior aspect of the arm, hands, and axillary fossa.

Pathology

Channel Pathology from the Nei Jing

The Heart Channel dominates the disorders of the heart. If the Heart Channel is disordered, there will be symptoms of **Bi Jue Syndrome** *(Abnormality of the arm)*. Symptoms include cardiac pain, dry throat, and thirst with desire to drink. There may also be yellow sclera, pain in the hypochondriac region, pain on the medial aspect of the arm, cold hands, and hot and painful palms.

Summary of Channel Pathology

Dominates Disorders Of	Heart
Channel Disorders	• <u>Channel Obstruction</u>: pain, swelling, hot or cold sensation on the medial aspect of the arm, palm, hypochondriac region, scapula, axillary fossa, chest and upper back. • <u>Heat Syndrome</u>: hot sensation of the body, hot flashes, night sweating, red face, thirst with desire to drink, dry throat. • <u>Eye Disorders</u>: redness, swelling of the eyes (especially the inner canthus), yellow sclera.
Organ Disorders	• <u>Heart and Lung</u>: cardiac pain, chest pain, palpitations, irregular heart beat, restlessness, shortness of breath. • <u>Mental and Emotional</u>: mental abnormality, insomnia, dream-disturbed sleep, sudden fainting, hysteria, shallow breathing. • <u>Digestive Disorders</u>: esophagitis, hiatal hernia.

The Clinical Applications

The Heart Channel is mainly used for the disorders of the heart and chest, mental and emotional disorders, and symptoms related to internal heat.

Category	Examples of Symptoms and Signs	Key points in order of importance.	Combinations with points from other channels.
Heart and Lung Disorders	Cardiac pain, palpitations, chest stuffiness, pain and pressure that refers to the upper extremities or throat, tachycardia, bradycardia, arrhythmia, shortness of breath, cold limbs, sweating, red, purple or pale complexion.	Ht 6, 5, 7	Pc 4, 6, 7, UB 15, Ren 17, SI 11

The Clinical Applications (continued)

Category	Examples of Symptoms and Signs	Key points in order of importance.	Combinations with points from other channels.
Mental, Emotional and Nervous System Disorders	Mental: manic-depression, schizophrenia, syncope.	Ht 7, 6, 4, 8	Pc 7, selection from 13 Ghost Points
	Nervous: nervousness, insomnia, restlessness, shallow breathing, muscle tension, spasm of the internal organs, dry mouth or throat, concentration difficulties, scattered thinking.	Ht 7, 4, 5	Pc 6, 7, Lv 3, GB 34, Ki 4 Ren 17
	Emotional: anxiety, hysteria, laughing or crying without apparent reason, mood swings.	Ht 7, 3, 5	Lv 3, Pc 6, LI 4, Du 11, Du 24
Heat Syndromes	Hot sensation of the body, dry mouth, yellow urination, red face, hot flashes with sweating, ulceration of the tongue, skin itching, boils, sunstroke.	Ht 3, 8, 7, 5	Ki 6, Ki 7, Pc 7, SI 2, LI 11
Eye Disorders	Redness, pain and/or swelling of the eyes (particularly the inner and outer canthi), yellow sclera.	Ht 5, 9, 3	Pc 9, Lv 2, Lv 3, LI 11, Taiyang
Painful Syndromes	Severe pain or spasm of the internal organs, post-traumatic or post-surgical pain, pain due to cancer.	Ht 7, 6	St 9, Lv 3, LI 4
Skin Disorders	Rashes, itching, pain of the skin, furuncles, carbuncles.	Ht 3, 7, 8	LI 11, LI 4, Sp10, Sp 6
Channel Disorders	Muscular pain of the chest and upper back, hypochondriac region, axillary fossa, medial aspect of the arm and palm.	Ht 2, 3, 7, 8	Pc 6, Ren 17, Lv 3, UB 15, SI 11

The Heart Divergent Channel

Pathway

After separating from the Heart Regular Channel at the axillary fossa (Ht 1 area), the Heart Divergent Channel enters the chest and connects with the heart. From there, it goes upward to the throat, emerges at the face, and finally converges with the Small Intestine Regular Channel at the inner canthus.

Separates from	Axillary fossa (Ht 1 area)
Enters the body cavity at	Chest
Connects with	Heart, throat, inner canthus
Emerges at	Face
Converges with the Small Intestine Regular channel at	Inner canthus

Clinical Applications

The Heart Divergent Channel further reinforces the connection between the Heart and the chest, further indicating that Heart Channel mainly focuses on treating heart and chest disorders. It does not connect with the small intestine.

The Divergent Channel's connection to the throat provides the rationale for choosing Heart points for disorders of the throat and vocal cords, such as laryngitis, pharyngitis, hoarseness, and aphonia. Points often used include Ht 5 and Ht 8, in combination with LI 4, Lu 7, St 40, and Ki 6.

The Divergent Channel establishes the connection between the Heart and the inner canthus. This supports the Five Wheel Theory's assertion that Heart disorders may be diagnosed from the canthus of the eye, and Heart points may be selected for disorders of the canthus. Points often used are Ht 5, Ht 8, and Ht 9 in combination with UB 1, SI 4, and SI 7.

The Heart Tendinomuscular Channel

- Starts from: Small finger (Ht 9 area)
- Ends at: Umbilicus
- Qi accumulates at: Wrist (Ht 7), elbow (Ht 3), axillary fossa, breast, chest, diaphragm, and umbilicus.

Pathway

From the small finger, the Heart Tendinomuscular Channel goes to the wrist and **knots** at the pisiform bone. It then travels up the forearm, and **knots** at the medial aspect of the elbow joint (Ht 3). It then continues upward and enters the axillary fossa, meeting the Lung Tendinomuscular Channel. After that it goes to the breast and **knots** in the middle of the chest, then passes through the diaphragm, and connects with the umbilicus.

Pathology

1. Stiffness, pulling, spasm, pain along the course of the Heart Tendinomuscular Channel.
2. Internal cramping near the heart area, which can be from disorders which produce angina-like symptoms, such as anxiety, hiatal hernia, and stomach disorders.

Clinical Applications

The primary applications of the Heart Tendinomuscular Channel are the treatment of pain, spasm, and hot sensation of the palm, small finger, ulnar side of the wrist, elbow, and shoulder joint. Since the Tendinomuscular Channel goes to the chest and breast, it can also be used for pain and constriction of the chest and breast, mastitis and fibrocystic breast disorders. Ht 3, Ht 7, and Ht 5 are often used in combination with Pc 6, St 40, and Ren 17.

The Tendinomuscular Channel passes through the diaphragm, indicating its use in such disorders as hiccups, belching, and esophagitis. Ht 3 and Ht 5 are often used in combination with Pc 6, Ren 14, and UB 17. It also connects with the umbilicus, which indicates that the Heart Channel has a direct connection to the Yuan (Source) Qi. When the Heart (mind) is shocked (as in syncope, fainting, coma, and sunstroke), applying moxibustion to the umbilicus (Ren 8) has a resuscitating effect.

The Luo Collateral of Heart Channel

Luo point: Ht 5
Distribution: After separating from the Heart Regular Channel, the Luo Collateral immediately goes to the Small Intestine Channel. It then follows the Heart Regular Channel until it reaches the heart, then goes to connect with the root of the tongue, and further to the eye system.
Connection: Heart, pericardium, eyes, root of tongue, Small Intestine Channel.

Pathology

<u>Excess:</u>   Distention and fullness in the chest and diaphragm

<u>Deficiency:</u>   Aphasia, disorders of the vocal cords

Clinical Applications

Chest and Diaphragm Disorders

Ht 5 is effective in treating cardiac pain, chest pain and stuffiness, anxiety, cough, and shortness of breath due to such disorders as angina pectoris, myocardial infarction, bronchitis, pneumonia, and emphysema. Points used in combination with Ht 5 are Pc 6, Pc 4, SI 4, Ren 17, UB 15, and UB 17.

Disorders of the Tongue and Vocal Cords

Ht 5 can be used for all types of tongue disorders including post-stroke[1] or post-traumatic aphasia. It can also be used for loss of voice, nodules and polyps on the vocals cords, laryngitis, and pharyngitis. Points used in combination with Ht 5 are St 40, St 9, LI 18, Ren 22, Ki 6, Lu 7, Lv 3.

Heart Fire Shifting to the Small Intestine

In the case of a red tongue tip with ulceration, irritability, burning, painful and concentrated urination, Ht 5 can be effectively used in combination with St 39, UB 39, and Ren 3.

---

[1] This is due to Phlegm misting the heart and heart being connected to the tongue.

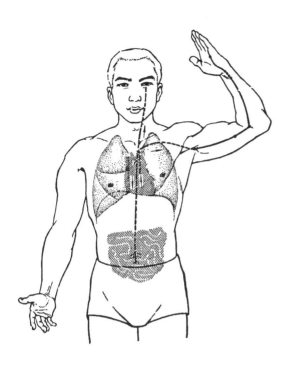

Heart Regular Channel

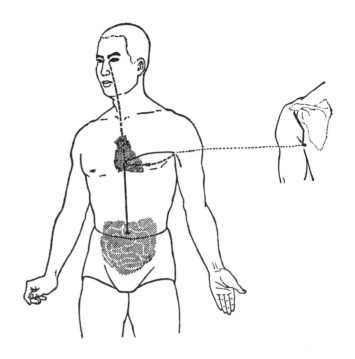

Heart Divergent Channel (---)
Small Intestine Divergent Channel (—)

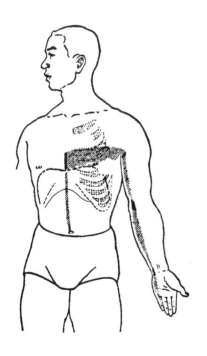

Heart Tendinomuscular Channel

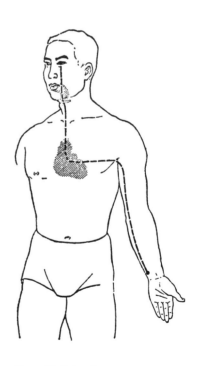

Heart Collateral

The Heart Channel of Hand-Shaoyin
手 少 陰 心 經 系 統 分 布 圖

6. The Small Intestine Channel of Hand - Tai Yang

手 太 陽 小 腸 經

Key Points

- The Small Intestine Channel starts at the ulnar side of the small finger (SI 1).
- The channel ends at the inner canthus and connects with the Urinary Bladder Channel (UB 1).
- It distributes mainly on the lateroposterior aspect of the arm, shoulder, scapular region, neck, face, ear, and the inner and outer canthi.
- It connects with the small intestine and heart.
- There are 19 points altogether.

The Pathway of the Small Intestine Regular Channel

External Pathway

The channel starts at the ulnar side of the small finger, then follows the ulnar side of the hand and wrist, going up to the lateroposterior aspect of the elbow. From there, it continues along the posterior aspect of the upper arm to the shoulder, where it curves around the scapular region (intersects UB 41) before reaching the upper back and neck intersects (UB 11 and Du 14). From Du 14, it goes to the supraclavicular fossa, where the channel bifurcates.

One branch enters the body cavity to begin the inner pathway. The other continues upward, along the neck, to the cheek, to the outer canthus (intersects GB 1 and SJ 22), and finally enters the ear. Another branch separates from the cheek. It passes through the lower border of the zygoma, and goes up along the lateral side of the nose to the inner canthus (intersects UB 1), where it connects with the Urinary Bladder Channel.

Internal Pathway

From the supraclavicular fossa, the main branch enters the body cavity and connects with the heart (intersects Ren 17). It then follows the sides of the esophagus, passes through the diaphragm, and goes to the stomach. It continues downward (intersects Ren 13 and Ren 12 on a deep level), then pertains to the small intestine. According to Chapter 4, "Pathogenic Qi and Zang Fu", of the Nei Jing Ling Shu (Spiritual Axis), there is a branch from the small intestine that descends to St 39, the Lower He (Sea) point of Small Intestine Channel.

The Associated Organs and Points

Pertains to	Connects with	Associated With	Intersecting Points
Small Intestine	Heart	Stomach, esophagus, diaphragm, ears, eyes, inner and outer canthi.	UB 41, UB 11, Du 14, GB 1, SJ 22, UB 1, Ren 17, Ren 13, Ren 12

Physiology

The Small Intestine Channel has the following functions:

1. *Distribute Qi to the face and head, and normalize the function of the ears and eyes.* This is the primary function. Symptoms such as deafness, ear ache, swelling and pain of the mandible and face,

pain of the inner and outer canthi, and yellow sclera implicate a disorder of the Small Intestine Channel.

2. *Distribute and regulate Qi along the channel pathway.* This especially applies to the neck and nape, upper back, scapular region, shoulder, arm, and ulnar side of the hands.

3. *Distribute Qi to the surface and strengthen the defensive functions of the body.* Since the Tai Yang Channels dominate the surface of the body, the Small Intestine Channel can be used for treatment of Exterior Syndromes.

4. *Regulate the body fluids (Ye).* According to Chapter 10, "Chapter of Channels" of the Nei Jing Ling Shu (Spiritual Axis), the Small Intestine Channel dominates the disorders of body fluids, called *Ye*. The Small Intestine Channel has an influence on the circulation of body fluids, and can be used for such symptoms as edema and concentrated, yellow urination.

5. *Regulate the function of the intestines and promote the absorption of fluids and nutrients.* Symptoms such as diarrhea, constipation, and abdominal distention implicate a disorder of the Small Intestine Channel. The Lower He (Sea) point (St 39) is often used.

6. *Regulate the Qi of the Lower Jiao.* Hernia, distention, pain, or cold sensation of the lower abdomen, which may refer to the lower back, testicles, or inguinal groove, may suggest a disorder of the Small Intestine Channel.

Pathology

Channel Pathology from the Nei Jing

The Small Intestine Channel dominates the disorders of *Ye*. If Qi in the channel is obstructed, there will be sore throat, swelling and pain of the mandible and cheek, pain of the nape of the neck which causes difficulty turning the head from side to side (lateral rotation), and pulling pain on the shoulder and the arm feels as if it is breaking (like being bent). Other symptoms include deafness, yellow sclera, and pain, numbness, cold or hot sensation which may occur on the scapula, shoulder, posterior aspect of the arm, elbow, and small finger.

Summary of Channel Pathology

Dominates Disorders Of	Ye (body fluids)
Channel Disorder	• Head, face, and sense organs: swelling and pain of the mandible and cheek, including TMJ syndrome, deafness, tinnitus, mumps, toothache, lymph gland swelling, sore throat (sides of throat), redness and pain of the eyes and canthi, yellow sclera, excessive lacrimation, mouth and tongue sores. • Exterior Syndrome: aversion to cold, fever, sweating or absence of sweating, general aching, headache. • Channel Obstruction: stiffness and pain of the neck and nape, restricted lateral rotation of the neck, pain along the channel distribution including the scapula, upper back, shoulder, arm, and hand. • Heat Syndrome: febrile diseases, fever, night sweating, yellow urination.

Summary of Channel Pathology (continued)

Organ Disorder[1]	• Body Fluid disorders: yellow urination, retention of urine, edema. • Digestive disorders: diarrhea, constipation, stomach pain, abdominal pain and distention • Qi obstruction in the Lower Jiao: distending pain in the lateral lower abdomen, referring to the lumbar region or testicles, inguinal hernia.

The Clinical Applications

The points of the Small Intestine Channel are mainly used for treating disorders of the head, face, Body Fluids, and channel disorders. Because the three Yang channels of the hand start from the hand and go to the face and head, their treatment strategies focus mainly on channel disorders. Their Fu organ disorders are generally treated by their Lower He (Sea) points.

Category	Examples of Symptoms and Signs	Key points in order of importance.	Combinations with points from other channels.
Head, face and sense organ disorders	Head: Occipital headache.	SI 3, 2	UB 10, UB 62, UB 65
	Ear: Deafness, swelling and pain of the ears, tinnitus.	SI 3, 2, 19, 6	SJ 2, SJ 3, GB 41, Ki 6
	Eye: Redness, swelling and pain of the inner and outer canthi, blurring of vision, excessive lacrimation, yellow sclera.	SI 6, 2, 1, 4, 3	Lv 2, Ht 5, UB 1, Tai Yang, Du 9, Lv 3, GB 37
	Mouth and tongue: sores, ulcerations, toothache.	SI 2, 3, 4, 7	Sp 2, LI 4, St 4, Pc 8
	Face and Throat: Swelling and pain of the cheek, lymph glands, parotid glands, mumps, TMJ syndrome.	SI 2, 3, 4, 7, 16, 17	LI 4, SJ 3, SJ 10, SJ 17, St 6, St 7
Exterior Syndrome	Wind Heat or Wind Cold (common cold, influenza).	SI 3, 7, 2	UB 12, Du 14, UB 65, LI 11, LI 4
	Allergic symptoms.	SI 3, 7	LI 11, LI 4, Lu 7, UB 12, UB 58
Heat Syndrome	Febrile diseases, fever, yellow. urination, night sweating.	SI 2, 3, 7	LI 11, Du 14, Ki 7
Channel Disorders	Pain and swelling of the scapula, shoulder, elbow, arm, wrist and small finger.	SI 10, 11, 14, 7, 5, 2, 3	St 39, St 38, SJ 5, LI 11, UB 62
	Neck: pain, stiffness, and restricted lateral rotation.	SI 3, 4, 6	UB 62, UB 65, Ht 4, UB 10
	Lower back pain	SI 6, 3	UB 40, UB 62
Body Fluid Disorders	Edema, retention of urine, painful and yellow urination.	SI 7, 3	Ren 3, St 39, Ht 5, Sp 9

---

[1] Zang/Fu disorders are not mentioned in Chapter 10, "Chapter of Channels", of the Nei Jing Ling Shu (Spiritual Axis). This information comes mainly from Nei Jing Su Wen (Plain Questions).

The Clinical Applications (continued)

Category	Examples of Symptoms and Signs	Key points in order of importance.	Combinations with points from other channels.
Digestive Disorders	Diarrhea, stomach pain, indigestion, abdominal pain and distention, constipation.	SI 3, 8	St 39, Ren 4, St 25, Sp 4, Pc 6
Stagnation of Qi in the Lower Jiao	Pain of the lateral lower abdomen referring to the back and testicles, such as inguinal hernia, epididymitis, orchitis, urethral stones, ovarian cysts, adnexitis.	SI 3, 7, 8	St 39, Lv 5, St 28, UB 27, Sp 6, UB 32

The Small Intestine Divergent Channel

Pathway

After separating from the Small Intestine Regular Channel at the shoulder (SI 10 area), the Divergent Channel goes to the axillary fossa, then enters the body cavity, connecting with the heart and small intestine.

Summary

Separates at	Shoulder (SI 10 area)
Enters the body cavity at	Axillary fossa (Ht 1)
Connects with	Heart, small Intestine
Emerges from	None
Converges with Small Intestine Regular Channel at	None

Clinical Applications

The Small Intestine Divergent Channel reinforces the relationship between the small intestine and the heart, providing a further theoretical basis for using the points of the Small Intestine Channel to treat disorders of the Heart Channel, and vice versa. An example of this is Heart Fire shifting to the Small Intestine, which results in dream-disturbed sleep, a red tongue or tongue ulcers, restlessness, and burning, yellow, and unsmooth urination. Small Intestine points such as SI 4 and SI 7 can be used in combination with Ht 5 and Sp 6.

Because the Small Intestine Divergent Channel enters the body cavity at SI 10, the energetic influence of this point directly facilitates the transportation of Qi to the Heart and Small Intestine. The pathological condition of those internal organs is often reflected as tenderness, swelling, or a depression at SI 10. In this case, SI 10 can be used to treat diarrhea, indigestion, and abnormal urination, in combination with St 39 (contralaterally), and Ren 4. It can also be used for treatment of chest pain, palpitations, and hypertension, in combination with Pc 6, Ht 7, SI 11, and St 36.

The Small Intestine Channel enters the body cavity at the axillary fossa (Ht 1). If there is swelling or pain of the axilla, it may be due to stagnation and accumulation of heat toxin transferring from the areas of the face and neck which are related to the Small Intestine Channel. Treatment for this disorder may include Ht 1 in combination with SI 2, SI 17, and SI 18.

The Small Intestine Tendinomuscular Channel

- Starts from: Ulnar side of the small finger.
- Ends at: Temporofrontal area of the head (St 8 area)
- Qi accumulates at: Ulnar side of the wrist and elbow, posterior aspect of the shoulder, axillary fossa, mastoid process, ear, mandible, outer canthus, and temporofrontal area.

Pathway
From the small finger, the Small Intestine Tendinomuscular Channel goes to the ulnar side of the wrist **(knots)**, along the forearm, and connects with the medial condyle of the humerus **(knots)**. From the elbow, it travels up the arm where it connects and **knots** at the posterior aspect of the axilla.

A branch separates from the posterior aspect of the axilla, circulates around the scapula, and then goes to the neck, **knots** behind the ear, and enters the ear. It emerges from the ear, travels down the face to the mandible **(knots)**, then ascends to the outer canthus **(knots)**.

Another branch separates from the mandible, goes upward and **knots** again at the outer canthus. From there it goes to the temporofrontal area, the place where the *three yang tendinomuscular channels of the hand knot and meet*.

Pathology
1. Stiffness, pulling, and pain of the small finger.
2. Pain of the medial condyle of the humerus (medial and posterior aspect).
3. Pain and pulling sensation in the axillary fossa, including the area below and on the posterior aspect.
4. Pain in the scapula referring to the neck or vice versa.
5. Tinnitus, pain in the ear referring to the mandible area.
6. Vision impairment.
7. Pain and spasm of the neck, or *Jing Lou*[1] (lymph gland swelling and pain, for example, cervical lymphadenopathy due to tuberculosis).
8. Stiffness and swelling of the neck due to invasion of cold or heat pathogen.

Clinical Applications
The Small Intestine tendinomuscular Channel treats tendinomuscular disorders along the channel distribution such as pain and spasm of the small finger, wrist, ulnar side of the elbow. It can also be used for the following:

As it covers the entire scapula region and m. trapezius, it treats muscle tension of the neck referring to the top of the shoulder and scapula, and vice versa. It is also effective for inflammation of the axillary fossa with referring pain to the arm, posterior aspect of the shoulder, or side of the chest. SI 6, SI 3, and SI 11 are often used in combination with Ht 3, Ht 1, LI 10, and SJ 8.

Both the Small Intestine Tendinomuscular and the Regular Channels enter the ear, emphasizing the use of Small Intestine points for ear pain which refers to the mandible or mastoid process (and vice versa). It can also be used for toothache referring to the ear or cheek. SI 4 and SI 5 are often used in combination with LI 6, SJ 17, and GB 41. Abnormal muscular contraction of the face, such as twitching of the eyelids, facial tic, and vision impairment can be treated by SI 6, SI 3, and SI 18 in combination with GB 1, Lv 3, and GB 37.

The Small Intestine Tendinomuscular Channel connects with the Large Intestine and San Jiao Tendinomuscular Channels at the temporofrontal area. Pain in that area (which may be due to eye disorders, migraine, or tension headache) can also be treated by SI 3 and SI 7, in combination with LI 4, SJ 8, SJ 5, and Lu 7.

---

[1] Jing Lou means "Lei Li" - swelling and pain of the lymph glands along the sides of the neck

The Luo Collateral of Small Intestine Channel

Luo point:	SI 7
Distribution:	After separating from the Small Intestine Regular Channel, the Luo Collateral goes immediately to the Heart Regular Channel, then travels to the medial condyle of the humerus. From there, it goes upward to the shoulder, making a network covering the whole shoulder area.
Connection:	Posteromedial aspect of the elbow and shoulder, and the Heart Channel.

Pathology

Excess:	Instability and weakness of the joints, weakness and paralysis of the elbow and arm.
Deficiency:	Flat warts[1]

Clinical Applications

Channel disorders

The Luo Collateral is used for Wei syndromes and weakness and instability of the joints, especially those of the entire upper extremity. Points used in combination with SI 7 are LI 15, LI 11, LI 4, and St 36.

Skin disorders

The original indication for flat warts comes directly from Chapter 10, "Chapter of Channels," of the Nei Jing Ling Shu (Spiritual Axis). Clinically, this can be extended to wide range of skin disorders such as rashes, hives, urticaria, herpes, psoriasis, eczema, and "liver spots." SI 7 is often used in combination with LI 11, Sp 10, LI 4, and Ht 7. A recently developed application for SI 7 is cosmetic skin treatments.

---

[1] This is a skin disorder which presents as many small growths with flat surfaces. This condition is usually due to a viral infection. These growths are light brown in color but do not involve pain or itching. They mainly grow on the face, neck and hands.

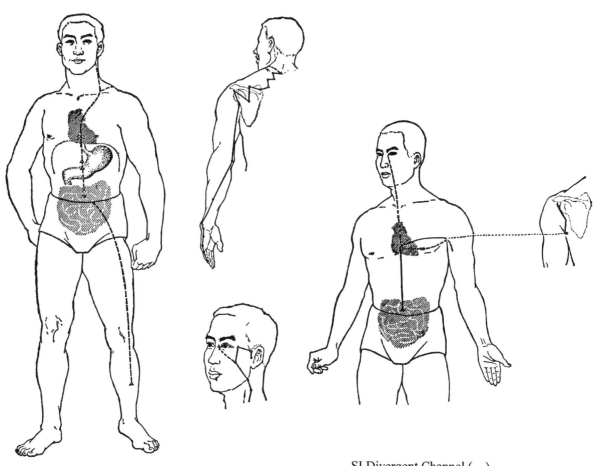

Small Intestine Regular Channel

SI Divergent Channel (—)
Heart Divergent Channel (---)

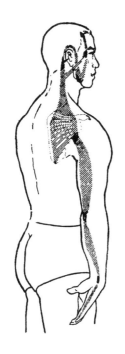

SI Tendinomuscular
Channel

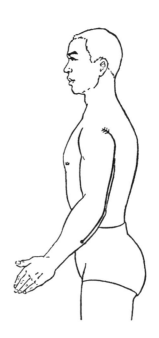

SI Collateral

The Small Intestine Channel of Hand-Taiyang
手 太 陽 小 腸 經 系 統 分 布 圖

7. The Urinary Bladder Channel of Foot - Tai Yang

足 太 陽 膀 胱 經

Key Points

- The Urinary Bladder Channel starts at the inner canthus (UB 1).
- The channel ends at the lateral aspect of the small toe (UB 67), connects with the Kidney Channel[1].
- It distributes mainly on the head, neck, back, posterior aspect of the lower extremities, and lateral aspect of the foot.
- It connects with the urinary bladder, kidney, and the Zang/Fu organs through their respective Back Shu points.
- There are 67 points altogether.

The Pathway of the Urinary Bladder Regular Channel

External Pathway

The channel begins at UB 1. It passes upward through the forehead (intersects Du 24 and GB 15), then goes toward the crown of the head, traveling 1.5 cun lateral to the midline, to the vertex (intersects Du 20). From there, it enters the brain. A branch descends laterally from the vertex, to the parietal area (intersects GB 6, GB7, GB 8, GB 10, GB 11, and GB 12).

The main pathway emerges from the brain at the nape (intersects Du 17, Du 16), and bifurcates. One branch travels down the nape of the neck, 1.5 cun lateral to the Du channel (intersects Du 14, Du 13). It continues down the back until it reaches the level of L 2, where it enters the body cavity. The external pathway continues to through the lumbar, sacral, and hip regions, then goes further down to the posterior aspect of the thigh, and enters the popliteal fossa.

The other branch travels down the back, 3 cun lateral to the Du channel. It goes down the back, passing by the medial border of the scapula, and continues until it reaches the gluteal area (intersects GB 30). It then follows the posterior aspect of the thigh to the popliteal fossa, where it meets the other branch. After the joining of the branches, the channel continues down the leg, through m. gastrocnemius to UB 60, then follows the lateral aspect of the foot, and ends at UB 67. Finally, it connects with the Kidney Channel on the inferior aspect of the small toe.

Internal Pathway

A branch from the vertex goes into the brain, then emerges at the nape area (Du 17). Another branch from the level of L 2 goes into the body cavity and connects with the kidney and urinary bladder. Through the Back Shu points, this channel connects with all the internal organs.

The Associated Organs and Points

Pertains to	Connects with	Associated With	Intersecting Points
Urinary bladder	Kidney	Brain, eye, heart[2]	Du 24, GB 15, Du 20, GB 6, GB 7, GB 8, GB 10, GB 11, GB 12, Du 17, Du 16, Du 14, Du 13, GB 30

---

[1] At the inferior aspect of the small toe.

[2] Through its divergent channel.

Physiology

The Urinary Bladder Channel has the following functions:

1. *Distribute Qi to consolidate the surface.* Tai Yang is considered the first line of defense against external invasion. It is related to the body's immunity. Symptoms such as chills, fever, body aches, headache, neck stiffness, and back pain may develop due to blocked Qi in the Tai Yang Channels.

2. *Circulate Qi to nourish the muscles and tendons.* The Urinary Bladder Channel has a strong energetic influence on, and promotes the functions of, the muscles, tendons, ligaments, and collagenous structures of the whole body. Symptoms such as tendinitis, muscular pain, injury and atony of the ligaments, and impaired movement of the muscles and joints may implicate a disorder of the Urinary Bladder Channel.

3. *Direct Qi to the brain to promote its functions and stabilize the emotions.* Symptoms such as Dian Kuang syndrome, epilepsy, manic-depression, schizophrenia, and emotional imbalances may suggest a disorder of the Urinary Bladder Channel.

4. *Distribute Qi to the sense organs and the head.* Symptoms such as headache in the occipital region, disorders of the eyes and nose, may result from stagnation of the Qi in the Tai Yang channel.

5. *Regulate the function of the Urinary Bladder and Kidney.* Symptoms such as retention of urine, enuresis, and male and female reproductive disorders, may result from impaired function of this channel.

6. Through the Back Shu points, the channel links with the Zang/Fu organs.

Pathology

Channel Pathology from the Nei Jing

The Urinary Bladder Channel dominates the disorders of tendons and ligaments. If the Urinary Bladder Channel is disordered, there will be ***Huai Jue Syndrome (Ankle Joint Disorder).*** Symptoms of this disorder include headache and a sensation of Qi rushing to the head (which may be accompanied by headache, or distending pain of the eyeball where the eyeball feels as it is falling out). Also included are painful nape and neck (where the neck feels like it is being pulled), back and lumbar pain (where the back feels as if it is being bent or breaking), inability to flex or extend the hip joint, spasm of the popliteal fossa, and splitting pain of the gastrocnemius muscle. There may also be Dian Kuang Syndrome, epilepsy, or mental disorders, pain of the fontanels, malaria, yellow sclera, excessive lacrimation, runny nose, epistaxis, hemorrhoids. Pain and impaired movement along the channel, nape, back, lumbar, sacrum, popliteal fossa, gastrocnemius, feet, and small toe may also occur.

According to Channel Theory, the Urinary Bladder Channel dominates disorders of the tendons and ligaments, while according to Zang/Fu Theory, it is the Liver which controls them. Clinically, both the Urinary Bladder and Liver Channels are used to treat these disorders. In order to differentiate this for clinically application, it should be noted that Urinary Bladder Channel is mainly applied to disorders of physical origin, such as Bi Syndrome and injury. The Liver Channel, which controls the emotions and nerves, is mainly used to treat muscle tightness or spasm due to nervous tension.

Summary of Channel Pathology

Dominates Disorders Of	Tendons, ligament, movement of muscles and joints
Channel Disorder	• <u>Channel obstruction</u>: pain, spasm and impaired movement of neck, nape, back, lumbar region, hip, knee, calf, leg, foot, and small toe. • <u>Exterior Syndromes</u>: chills, fever, headache, nape stiffness, runny nose, body aches, easily catching cold. • <u>Head, face and sense organs</u>: yellow sclera, painful eyes with lacrimation, obstruction of the nose, epistaxis.
Organ Disorder[1]	• <u>Urogenital system</u>: unsmooth urination with distention and pain of the lower abdomen, retention of urine, enuresis, dysmenorrhea, leukorrhea. • <u>Mental and emotional disorders</u>: Dian Kuang syndrome, epilepsy, depression, excessive worry, phobias, fears. • <u>Internal organs</u>: Chronic and deficient conditions of all internal organs.
Other Disorders	• Opisthotonos, malaria

The Clinical Applications

The points of the Urinary Bladder Channel are mainly applied for the disorders of the posterior aspect of the body, and for Tai Yang exterior syndromes. They are also used for Zang/Fu disorders, especially those of chronic or deficient natures, and mental and emotional disorders.

Category	Examples of Symptoms and Signs	Key points in order of importance	Combinations with points from other channels.
Disorders of Tendons, Ligaments, Muscles and Joints	<u>Pain</u>: Nape and neck pain <u>Bi Syndrome</u>: Upper back Lower back Sacrum and hip Posterior aspect of the lower extremities <u>Acute sprain or traumatic injury</u>: Neck, back, lumbar regions spinal column, and lower extremities	UB 62, 60, 65, 10 UB 57, 58, 17, 11 UB 40, 39, 58, 23, 25 UB 36, 40, 31, 32, 54 UB local points, 10 UB 40, 58, 2, 10, 54	SI 3, SI 4 SI 6, LI 10, 11, GB 34, Lv 3 SI 3, GB 34, St 36, Lv 6 St 32, GB 30, 29, 34, SJ 5, Lv 3 GB 34, St 36, Lv 3 Du 26, Yaotongdian, SI 3, SI 6, LI 4

---

[1] There were no internal organ symptoms in this chapter of the Nei Jing. These were add from other chapters.

The Clinical Applications (continued)

Category	Examples of Symptoms and Signs	Key points in order of importance	Combinations with points from other channels.
Exterior Syndrome	Wind Cold, Wind Heat (common cold, influenza)	UB 12, 10, 13, 38	LI 4, 11, SJ 5, Du 14
	Allergy (especially with lacrimation and runny nose)	UB 12, 10, 2, 7, 58	Du 14, St 36, LI 11, LI 4, Lu 7
Head, face and sense organ disorders	Occipital headache	UB 65, 60, 10	SI 3, SI 6, Ki 16
	Eye disorders: pain, lacrimation, optic nerve atrophy, glaucoma, retinitis, et al.	UB 1, 2, 7, 62, 66	Lv 3, GB 37, SI 6, LI 11, Ki 6
	Nose disorders: rhinitis, sinusitis, epistaxis, et al.	UB 58, 7, 10	LI 4, Lu 7, St 36, Sp 3, GB 40
Mental disorders	Manic-depression, schizophrenia	UB 62, 10, 15, 18	Selection from 13 Ghost Points
	Epilepsy	UB 62, 18	Du 2, Ren 15, Ki 6, SI 3
Emotional disorders (Dysfunction of *Five Zhi*)	Heart related: anxiety, excessive excitement, laughing or crying without apparent reason	UB 44, 15	Du 11, H 7, Pc 7, Pc 8
	Lung related: weeping, worry, sadness with restricted sense in the chest	UB 42, 13	Du 12, Lu 7, Ren 17
	Liver related: depression, anger, frustration, poor judgment	UB 47, 18, 19	Du 8, Lv 3, GB 34, Du 20
	Spleen related: melancholia, obsessive thinking, worry	UB 49, 20	Sp 3, Sp 4, Pc 6
	Kidney related: fear, fright, depression, lack of will power	UB 52, 23	Du 4, Ki 3, Ki 6, UB 62
Urogenital disorders	Urinary Bladder Disorders: painful, unsmooth urination, retention of urine, enuresis, kidney and urinary bladder stones	UB 28, 32, 39, 58, 23	Ren 3, Sp 9, Sp 6, Ki 3
	Gynecological Disorders: irregular menstruation, dysmenorrhea, infertility, PMS, leukorrhea, malposition of fetus, adnexitis, et al.	UB 23, 32, 60, 9, 10, 67	Du 3, Lv 3, Lv 5, Sp 6, Ki 6, Ren 4, St 28, St 29, Zigong, GB 28
	Male Reproductive Disorders: prostatitis, impotence, nocturnal emission, spermatorrhea	UB 33, 34, 26, 23, 40, 58, 62	Ren 1, Ren 4, Ki 3, Sp 6, Lv 8, St 36
Disorders of Zang/Fu organs	Symptoms and signs of every organ, especially chronic or deficient conditions.	Back Shu points	Front Mu and Yuan (Source) points of associated organs
Other disorders	Opisthotonos	UB 62, 44, 15	Du 14, Du 1, Du 16, SI 3
	Malaria	UB 11, 12, 13, 62	Du 13, Pc 5

The Urinary Bladder Divergent Channel

Pathway

After separating from the Regular Channel at the popliteal fossa, the Urinary Bladder Divergent Channel goes up to the sacrum (5 sun above the anus), approximately the area of UB 31. From there, two branches diverge. One branch goes to the anus. A second branch goes internally to connect with the urinary bladder, then disperses to the kidney, then up to connect with the heart. The main pathway continues upward through the muscles along side the spinal column, and emerges at the nape where it converges with the Urinary Bladder Regular Channel.

Summary

Separates at	Popliteal fossa (UB 40 area)
Enters the body cavity at	5 cun above the anus
Connects with	Urinary bladder, kidney, heart, anus
Emerges from	Nape, (UB 10 area)
Converges with the Urinary Bladder Regular Channel at	Nape (UB 10 area)

Clinical Applications:

The Urinary Bladder Divergent Channel reinforces the relationship between the Urinary Bladder and the Kidney, supporting the use of Urinary Bladder points for disorders of the Kidney, and vice versa. The Divergent Channel establishes a connection between the Urinary Bladder Channel, the anus, and rectal area. Clinically, we can use UB 57, UB 40, and UB 35, for hemorrhoids and prolapse of the rectum.

Urinary Bladder Divergent Channel is connected with the heart. When the Heart's function of Housing the Mind is disturbed, there may be urinary disorders related to nervousness, such as frequency and urgency to urinate with little volume. In these cases, UB 28 and UB 23 can be used effectively in combination with Ht 7 and Lv 3. When the fire of the heart flares up, causing yellow, scanty, burning urination, or enuresis, we can treat with Urinary Bladder points, such as UB 58, UB 66, and UB 33.

UB 40 and UB 10 are the separating and converging points, respectively, of the Divergent Channel. This indicates a specific connection between the two areas. Clinically, both points can be used to treat pain and stiffness of the nape and neck, as well as pain of the knee joint, popliteal fossa, and m. gastrocnemius.

The sacral region is also related to the nape through the Divergent Channel, indicating that point on the sacrum, such as UB 32 and 31, can be used to treat neck pain. Neck area points can also be applied for disorders of the sacral area. This connection should be further understood to include a relationship between the nape and the pelvic region. Clinically, UB 10 can be used for gynecological disorders due to hormonal imbalance, such as irregular menstruation, dysmenorrhea, infertility, and PMS.

The Urinary Bladder Tendinomuscular Channel

- Starts from: Small toe
- Ends at: Nose
- Qi accumulates at: External malleolus, heel, knee, popliteal fossa, gluteal region, back, nape, root of the tongue, nose, eyelid, scapula, shoulder, mastoid process.

Pathway

From the small toe, a branch of the Urinary Bladder Tendinomuscular Channel goes to the external malleolus, approximately GB 40 **(knots)**, then up to the lateral aspect of the knee **(knots)**. The main pathway goes from the small toe to the lateral aspect of the heel **(knots)**. From there, it follows the calcaneal tendon to m. gastrocnemius where it bifurcates. One branch goes to the center of the popliteal fossa (approximately UB 40), and **knots** there. The other goes to the area of UB 39 and **knots**. The main pathway continues on the posterior aspect of the thigh to the gluteal region **(knots)**, then up along side the spinal column to the occiput and the nape **(knots)**. A branch from the nape goes internally, connecting with the *root of the tongue* **(knots)**.

The main pathway continues over the head and down the forehead, where it **knots** at the nose. A branch from the nose *connects with the upper eyelid*, then goes back to the side of the nose, where it **knots** again. From the major pathway on the back (at about the level of the inferior angle of the scapula), there are two branches. One passes through the scapula to the shoulder, and **knots** (around LI 15). The other goes under the arm to the axillary fossa, then to the supraclavicular fossa, and further up to the mastoid process **(knots)**. From the supraclavicular fossa, a branch goes to the face and **knots** beside the nose.

Pathology

1. Strained muscles of the small toe.
2. Swelling and pain in the heel.
3. Spasms and stiffness of the joints.
4. Spasm and stiffness of the back or along the sides of the spine causing difficulty in bending forward.
5. Inability to raise the arm at the shoulder.
6. Stiffness or pulling sensation in the axillary region.
7. Pain and strained muscles at the supraclavicular fossa.
8. Impaired rotation of the neck.

Clinical Application:

The Urinary Bladder Tendinomuscular Channel treats tendinomuscular disorders along the channel distribution, such as pain and spasm of the small toe, foot, ankle, posterior and lateral aspect of the lower extremities, hip, back, and nape. It can also be used for the following:

The Tendinomuscular Channel knots at the external malleolus, heel, mastoid process, and nape, indicating a specific connection between these upper and lower areas. Clinically, using UB 10 and GB 12 are very effective for ankle sprains and pain due to bone spurs in combination with local points. As it distributes on both the lateral and posterior aspects of the knee and thigh, Urinary Bladder points are indicated for knee pain involving both the lateral aspect and the popliteal fossa.

The Tendinomuscular Channel also circulates on the scapula, shoulder, axillary fossa, the supraclavicular fossa and upward from there to the mastoid process. That is why symptoms such as pain, spasm, stiffness, pulling sensation in those areas, inability to raise the arm at the shoulder, and difficult movement of the neck, can be treated by UB 60, UB 59, and UB 10. These points are often used in combination with SI 6, SI 3, SI 11, and LI 10. With the additional coverage added by the Tendinomuscular Channel's distribution to the scapula and shoulder, the Urinary Bladder Channel should be understood to dominate disorders of the entire back.

The Tendinomuscular Channel forms a network to connect with the upper eyelid, therefore Urinary Bladder points are useful for disorders such as blepharoptosis and inability to close the eyes due to Bell's palsy. The channel knots at the nose three times, reinforcing the theoretical basis for applying Urinary Bladder points such as UB 58, UB 7, and UB 2 for nose disorders. It is also connected to the tongue. Since this connection is established through UB 10, this point is clinically effective for tongue, throat, and thyroid disorders.

Since the Tendinomuscular Channel distributes on the sides of the chest, the axillary fossa, and neck, Urinary Bladder points are also useful for lymph swellings of the axillary fossa and neck, and for pain on the lateral side of the breast and chest. It also treats referred pain, and muscle strain in these areas due to liver and gall bladder disorders, and ear ache.

The Luo Collateral of Urinary Bladder Channel

Luo point:	UB 58.
Distribution:	After separating from the Urinary Bladder Regular Channel, the Luo Collateral goes immediately to and connects with the Kidney Regular Channel.
Connection:	Kidney Channel.

Pathology

Excess:	Nasal obstruction, clear nasal discharge, headache, back pain.
Deficiency:	Epistaxis, chronic clear nasal discharge, sinusitis.

Clinical Applications

Exterior Syndrome

UB 58 is used for Wind Cold or Wind Heat syndromes manifesting with occipital headache, stiffness of the neck, nasal obstruction, nasal discharge, body aches, and back pain. It is also used for similar symptoms due to allergy. Points used in combination with UB 58 are Lu 7, LI 4, UB 12, St 37, and UB 38.

Disorders of the Nose

This point can be used in general for disorders of the nose, both excess and deficiency types. Some examples include rhinitis, sinusitis, epistaxis, and nasal polyps. Points used in combination with UB 58 are LI 4, Lu 7, LI 20, LI 11, UB 10, Bitong, and St 36.

Channel Disorders

This point is especially good for pain ranging from the middle to the lower back, due to Bi syndrome, or from muscle strain or trauma. Points used in combination with UB 58 are UB 57, SI 3, Ki 3, and GB 34.

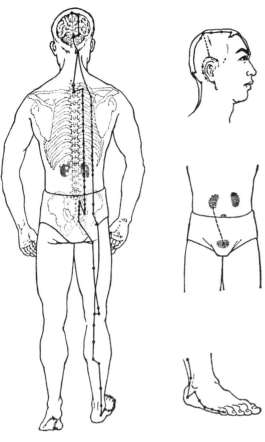
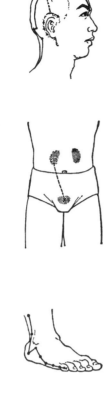
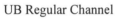

UB Regular Channel

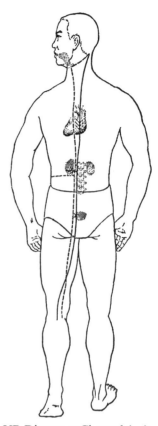

UB Divergent Channel (—)
Kidney Divergent Channel (---)

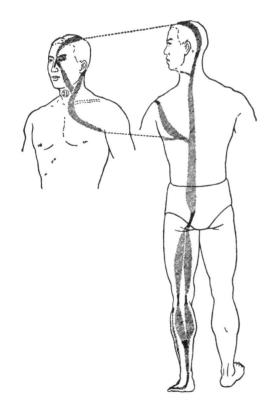

UB Tendinomuscular Channel

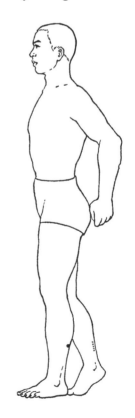

UB Collateral

The Urinary Bladder Channel of Foot-Taiyang
足 太 陽 膀 胱 經 系 統 分 布 圖

8. The Kidney Channel of Foot - Shao Yin

足 少 陰 腎 經

Key Points

- The Kidney Channel starts at the inferior aspect of the small toe.
- The channel ends at the chest, externally (Ki 27), and connects with the Pericardium Channel in the middle of the chest, internally.
- It distributes mainly on the medioposterior aspect of the lower extremities, spinal column, abdomen, chest, throat, and tongue.
- It connects with the kidney and urinary bladder, liver, lung, heart, and pericardium.
- There are 27 points altogether.

The Pathway of the Kidney Regular Channel

External Pathway

The Kidney Regular Channel begins at the inferior aspect of the small toe, goes to the sole of the foot, then to the medial aspect of the foot. From there, it curves around the medial malleolus, connects with the heel, then goes up the medioposterior aspect the lower leg (intersects Sp 6), knee, and thigh, to the tip of the coccyx (intersects Du 1). From Du 1, a branch goes to the symphysis pubis, 1.5 lateral to the midline of the lower abdomen (and a sub-branch intersects Ren 3 and 4). The main pathway continues up the abdomen. When it reaches the chest, its distance from the midline increases to 2 cun lateral. It travels all the way up the chest, and ends below the clavicle (Ki 27).

Internal Pathway

From the coccyx, the channel goes internally, running anterior to the spinal column. It then enters the body cavity, pertains to the kidney, and connects with the urinary bladder and the uterus. A branch goes from the kidney to the liver, and passes through the diaphragm to the Lung. It continues up along side the esophagus to the throat, connecting with the root of the tongue. A second branch is derived from the Lung and goes into the heart. It flows into the chest, and connects with the Pericardium Channel, where it ends.

The Associated Organs and Points

Pertains to	Connects with	Associated With	Intersecting Points
Kidney	Urinary bladder	Liver, lung, heart, pericardium, throat, tongue, and uterus	Sp 6, Du 1, Ren 3, Ren 4

Physiology

The Kidney Channel has the following functions:

1. *Circulate Kidney Qi and Essence.* It maintains the function of the kidneys, strengthen the bones and lumbar region. It promotes the reproductive function and the circulation of body fluids. Symptoms such as back pain, pain along the spinal column, pain and hot sensations of the sole of the foot, weakness of the lower extremities, male and female reproductive disorders, brain disorders, poor memory, edema, and urinary dysfunction suggest disorders of the Kidney Channel.

2. *Promote the function of the stomach and spleen.* Symptoms such as hunger without desire to eat and chronic diarrhea, implicate deficiency of Kidney Qi.
3. *Promote the function of the lung and heart.* Symptoms such as shortness of breath, asthmatic breathing, chronic cough with hemoptysis, restlessness, anxiety, and being easily frightened, suggest lung and heart disorders due to deficiency of Kidney Qi.
4. *Promote the function of the liver.* Dizziness, vertigo, dark and withered complexion, and blurring of vision, suggest a deficiency of Kidney Qi as the root cause of the liver disorder.
5. *Promote the function of the throat and tongue.* Symptoms such as chronic throat and vocal cord disorders, and dry or painful tongue and throat, may indicate a disorder of Kidney Channel.

Pathology

Channel Pathology from the Nei Jing

The Kidney Channel dominates the disorders of the Kidney. If the Kidney Channel is disordered, there will be hunger with no desire to eat, a dark and withered complexion, cough or hemoptysis, asthmatic breathing[1], blurred vision, and palpitations. There will also be anxiety, such that the heart feels as if it is out of its place. This gives a sense of uneasiness, similar to being hungry.

When the Qi of the channel is deficient, **Gu Jue Syndrome *(Bone Abnormality)*** may develop. Symptoms include being easily frightened or fearful, and experiencing palpitations, as if being chased. There may also be dry tongue, hot sensation in the mouth, swollen and dry throat, shortness of breath, a sensation of Qi rushing upward to the chest and head, restlessness, cardiac pain, somnolence, jaundice, diarrhea, pain along the medioposterior aspect of the lower extremities and spinal column, muscular atrophy, coldness of the lower limbs, and a hot sensation and pain of the sole of the foot.

Summary of Channel Pathology

Dominates Disorders Of	Kidney
Channel Disorder	• <u>Channel deficiency and obstruction</u>: pain and weakness of the lower back, knee joint, spinal column, hip, and medioposterior aspect of the lower extremities, degenerative disorders of the bones and joints, Wei Syndrome, cold, pain, or heat of the sole of the feet. • <u>Throat and tongue</u>: dry mouth and tongue, chronic sore throat.
Organ Disorder	• <u>Kidney and urinary bladder</u>: edema, facial puffiness, impotence, infertility, forgetfulness. • <u>Kidney and liver</u>: dizziness, blurred vision, dark circles and puffiness under the eyes, dark and withered complexion, or darkening of the skin (like liver spots). • <u>Kidney and spleen/stomach</u>: loose stools, chronic diarrhea or constipation, abdominal distention, hunger with no desire to eat, vomiting, nausea. • <u>Kidney, heart and lung</u>: restlessness, insomnia or somnolence, palpitations, cardiac pain, anxiety, a sensation of Qi rushing upward to the chest and head, shortness of breath, labored breathing, chronic cough with hemoptysis.
Qi Deficiency	• Being easily fatigued, fear, anxiety, easily frightened resulting in palpitations as if being chasing.

---

[1] This is a type of asthmatic breathing due to the Kidney being unable to grasp the Qi. The person is unable to lie down flat, can't sit and wants to stand up, i.e. uneasiness. If they sit they make a loud wheezing sound.

The Clinical Applications

The points of the Kidney Channel are mainly used for disorders of the kidney. Since the kidney is the root of the Zang/Fu organs, kidney points may be used for chronic disorders of the other organs.

Category	Examples of Symptoms and Signs	Key points in order of importance	Combinations with points from other channels.
Kidney Deficiency	• Qi: easily fatigued, lower back pain, pain of the spinal column, muscular atrophy.	Ki 3, 4, 6	UB 23, Du 4, Ren 4, Ren 6
	• Essence: poor memory, forgetfulness, hair loss, chronic tooth and gum disorders, tinnitus, deafness	Ki 3, 6	UB 23, GB 39, Kidney Essence point[1], Du 20, Ht 7
	• Yin: hot sensation and pain of the sole and heel, dry mouth and tongue, thirst, chronic sore throat, hot flashes, night sweating.	Ki 2, 6, 7	Sp 6, Lu 7, Ht 5, UB 52
	• Yang: cold feet and hands, cold appearance, curling up the body.	Ki 3, 7, 6	UB 23, Ren 4, Du 4, UB 62
Reproductive disorders	• Male: impotence, nocturnal emission, premature ejaculation, spermatorrhea.	Ki 3, 6, 11	UB 23, Du 3, Du 4, UB 31, Sp 6, Ren 4
	• Female: irregular menstruation, functional uterine bleeding, infertility, leukorrhea.	Ki 3, 6, 8, 7	UB 23, Du 4, Kidney Essence point, Sp 6, Lv 3
Kidney/Urinary Bladder disorders	• Edema, facial puffiness, abnormal urination, retention of urine, frequent urination (especially at night).	Ki 3, 7, 10, 6	Ren 4, Ren 9, Ren 3, UB 23, UB 28
Kidney/Liver Deficiency disorders	• Dizziness, tinnitus, headache with empty feeling in the head, blurring of vision, unclear vision, chronic glaucoma, optic nerve atrophy.	Ki 6, 3	Lv 3, Lv 8, GB 37, Du 20, UB 1, UB 2
	• Dark withered complexion, darkening of skin color, increased pigmentation, jaundice.	Ki 3, 9, 4	Du 4, UB 23, UB 19, Sp 10, Lv 3, Du 9
Kidney/Lung and Heart disorders	• Asthmatic breathing, shortness of breath, chronic cough with hemoptysis, difficulty breathing (inability to breath comfortably when lying down).	Ki 7, 6, 3	Ren 6, Ren 17, UB 23, UB 43, St 36
	• Restlessness, being easily frightened, palpitations, insomnia or somnolence, anxiety, fear, feeling as if being chased, sensation of Qi rushing upward.	Ki 4, 3, 6	Lu 7, Ht 7, Pc 6, UB 52, UB 15
Kidney/Spleen-Stomach disorders	• Hunger without desire to eat, chronic diarrhea or morning diarrhea, constipation, abdominal distention.	Ki 3, 6, 9	UB 23, Du 4, UB 20, UB 21, Ren 4, Ren 12

---

[1] Located three cun bilateral to the intervertebral space between L3 and L4.

The Kidney Divergent Channel

Pathway

The Kidney Divergent Channel is unusual in that it runs on the back, rather than the front of the body. After separating from the Regular Channel at the popliteal fossa (Ki 10 area), the Kidney Divergent Channel joins, and runs together with the Urinary Bladder Divergent Channel. At the second lumbar vertebra, a branch emerges to start the Dai channel. The main portion continues upward to the nape, where it both emerges and converges with the Urinary Bladder Regular Channel (UB 10 area). A branch from the nape goes to the root of the tongue.

Separates from	Popliteal fossa (Ki 10 area)
Enters the body cavity at	Same as Urinary Bladder Divergent Channel
Connects with	Kidney, urinary bladder, root of the tongue, Dai channel
Emerges from	Nape (UB 10 area)
Converges with the Urinary Bladder Regular Channel at	Nape (UB 10 area)

Clinical Applications

The Divergent Channel reinforces the relationship between the Kidney and Urinary Bladder, demonstrating that Kidney Channel points can be used to treat the disorders of the Urinary Bladder, and vice versa. By virtue of its connection with the Dai Channel, it can be used for such Dai Channel disorders. Some examples include leukorrhea, weakness and paralysis of the lumbar area and lower extremities, and pain and tightness of the groin and sacral regions which may refer to the lower extremities. Points often used are Ki 6 and Ki 3, in combination with Du 4 and GB 26.

The Kidney Divergent Channel distributes on the nape, and the Kidney Regular Channel is connected with the uterus. Clinically, the use of Ki 10 and UB 10 in combination with Du 4, or Ren 4, activates a flow of Qi, which links the kidney, uterus, and nape. When occipital headaches occur, along with a stiff and painful neck (and these symptoms develop around the time of menstruation or ovulation), Kidney Channel points, such as Ki 6, Ki 8, Ki 10, and Ki 16, can be effectively used, in combination with UB 10, UB 9, and UB 23.

The Divergent Channel sends the Kidney Qi and Essence directly to the brain through the spinal cord, establishing the connection between the kidney, marrow, spinal cord, and brain. Clinically, Kidney Channel points such as Ki 3 and Ki 6, are often selected for treating disorders of the brain and mind.

The Divergent Channel connects with the tongue, as does the Regular Channel. This second connect reinforces the selection of Kidney Channel points for aphasia, stiffness or flaccidity of the tongue, and speech difficulties. Ki 6 and Ki 10 are often used in combination with UB 10, Ren 23, and St 40.

The Kidney Tendinomuscular Channel

- Starts from: Inferior aspect of the small toe.
- Ends at: Nape.
- Qi accumulates at: Heel, medial aspect of the knee, external genitalia, and occiput.

Pathway

The Kidney Tendinomuscular Channel starts from the inferior aspect of the small toe. It follows the Regular Channel to the medial aspect of the foot, medial malleolus, and heel (**knots**), where it joins the Urinary Bladder Tendinomuscular Channel. It then goes up the leg to the medial aspect of the knee (**knots**), and upward

70

along the medial aspect of the thigh to the lateral side of the genital region **(knots)**. A branch from the genital area goes to the back and alongside the spine to the nape, where it connects with the occipital protuberance **(knots)**, and converges with the Urinary Bladder Tendinomuscular Channel.

Pathology

1. Spasm of the plantar aspect of the foot, plantar fascitis, and bone spurs.
2. Pain or spasm on the medioposterior aspect of the lower extremities, back, and nape. All types of chronic Bi syndrome.
3. Epilepsy, convulsion, trembling, twitching, and shivering
4. Difficulty bending forward and backward. This includes the neck, back, and lumbar area. If Kidney Yang is disordered, the patient cannot bend forward, if Kidney Yin is disordered the patient cannot bend backward.
5. Degeneration of bone and joints, spondylosis, osteoarthritis.

Clinical Applications

The primary function of the Kidney Tendinomuscular Channel is to treat chronic pain, spasm, and cold sensation on the lower back and spinal column, with difficulty in bending forward and backward. It is also used for treating these symptoms along the rest of channel distribution. This includes the posteromedial aspect of the lower extremities, the hamstring, and m. gastrocnemius. Clinically, Ki 3, Ki 4, and Ki 7 are often selected, in combination with UB 58, UB 40, and UB 23.

Kidney points can be used for foot pain due to bone spurs, plantar fascitis and burning sensation of the sole, because the Tendinomuscular Channel knots at the heel. The thenar eminence of the opposite hand is palpated for tenderness and needled first (with Miu Ci method), then a Kidney point is selected, such as Ki 2, Ki 5, or Ki 3, combined with UB 62.

Both the Kidney Tendinomuscular Channel and Divergent Channel go to the nape, and are further connected to the brain. This provides the theoretical basic for treating brain disorders such as epilepsy, convulsion, and trembling. Ki 4 and Ki 6 are generally used in combination with Du 16 and UB 10.

The Luo Collateral of Kidney Channel

Luo point: Ki 4
Distribution: After separating from the Kidney Regular Channel, the Luo Collateral bifurcates. One branch immediately connects with the Urinary Bladder Regular Channel. The other follows the Kidney Regular Channel to the area below the heart. It then goes inside the body cavity, to the back, then downward through the spinal column.
Connection: Epigastric region, spinal column, Urinary Bladder Channel.

Pathology

Excess: Retention of urine.
Deficiency: Lumbar pain.
Rebellious Qi: Restlessness, anxiety, fear, depression, stuffiness of the chest and epigastrium.

Clinical Applications

Channel disorders

Ki 4 can be used for chronic lower back pain due to arthritis and muscular strain and tension. It can also be used for disorders involving the entire spinal column, such as osteoarthritis and spondylosis, causing stiffness and pain of the back. Points used in combination with Ki 4 are UB 64, and UB23.

Organ disorders

The Luo point can be used for chronic urinary dysfunction such as enuresis, incontinence, and retention of urine. Points used in combination with Ki 4 are Ki 3, Du 4, UB 23, and Ren 4. It can also be used for epigastric disorders, especially for *Pi Zheng*[1], hiatal hernia, chronic gastritis, and peptic ulcer. Points used in combination with Ki 4 are Pc 6, St 36, Ren 10.

Emotional Disorders

This point has a strong effect on emotional disorders, and can be used to treat depression, anxiety and fear due to Kidney Qi rebellion or deficiency. The treatment requires tonifying Kidney Qi and Lifting the Spirit rather than regulating the Qi. Points used in combination with Ki 4 are Lu 7, Pc 6, Du 20, and UB 52.

---

[1] Distention and fullness sensation in the epigastrium due to non-substantial accumulation. It is a stagnation of Qi which is not painful with pressure. It is typically treated with Ban Xia Xie Xin Tang (Pinellia Decoction to Drain the Epigastrium).

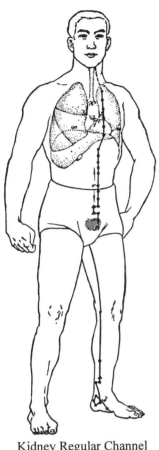
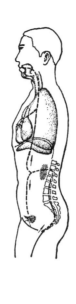

Kidney Regular Channel

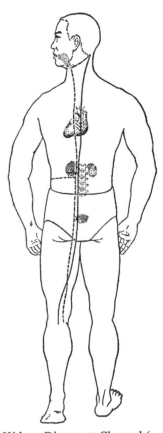

Kidney Divergent Channel (---)
UB Divergent Channel (—)

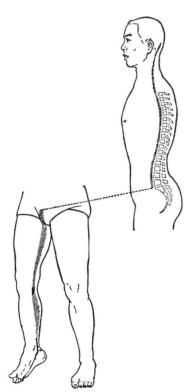

Kidney Tendinomuscular Channel

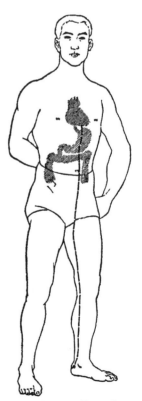

Kidney Collateral

The Kidney Channel of Foot-Shaoyin

足 少 陰 腎 經 系 統 分 布 圖

9. The Pericardium Channel of Hand - Jue Yin
手 厥 陰 心 包 經

Key Points
* The Pericardium Channel starts in the chest.
* The channel ends at the radial side of the fourth finger (SJ 1) where it connects with the San Jiao Channel.
* It distributes mainly on the chest, middle and lower abdomen, breast, anterior aspect of the axillary region, and medial aspect of the arm and hand.
* It connects with the pericardium and San Jiao.
* There are 9 points altogether.

The Pathway of the Pericardium Regular Channel

Internal Pathway
The Pericardium Regular Channel starts in the chest and connects with the pericardium. From there, it goes through the diaphragm and connects successively with each of the Three Jiaos. A branch from the chest goes laterally and emerges at Pc 1, which is three cun below the axillary fossa and one cun lateral to the nipple.

External Pathway
From Pc 1, the Regular Channel goes to the anterior aspect of the axillary fossa, then along the medial aspect of the upper extremities. It passes between the tendons m. palmaris longus and m. flexor radialis to the medial aspect of the wrist, then goes along the middle finger and ends at its tip. A branch separates from the middle of the palm, goes along the ring finger to SJ 1, where it ends.

The Associated Organs and Points

Pertains to	Connects with	Associated With	Intersecting Points
Pericardium	San Jiao	Breast	None

Physiology

The functions of the Pericardium Channel include many of those associated with the Heart Channel. It also exerts a special influence on the Upper and Middle Jiaos, i.e., the chest and stomach. Its functions are as follows:
1. *Regulate the vessels and blood circulation.* Symptoms such as palpitations, cardiac pain, coronary disease, and high lipid levels may suggest a disorder of the Pericardium Channel.
2. *Assist the Heart in Housing the Mind.* Symptoms such as restlessness, delirium, and incessant laughing may indicate a disorder of the Pericardium Channel.
3. *Maintain open flow of Qi in the chest.* Symptoms such as stiffness, stuffiness, suffocating sensation, or a restricted feeling in the chest, as well as shallow breathing, cough, asthma, and depression may suggest a disorder of the Pericardium Channel.

4. *Distribute Qi to, and regulate the function of the stomach and diaphragm.* Symptoms such as epigastric pain and distention, hiccup, nausea, and vomiting may implicate a disorder of Pericardium Channel.

5. *Distribute Qi to the areas covered by the Pericardium Channel.* This includes as the chest, abdomen, axillary area, and medial aspect of the arm and palm.

Pathology

Channel Pathology from the Nei Jing

The Pericardium dominates the disorders of the vessels. If the Pericardium Channel is disordered, there may be cardiac pain, restlessness, palpitations, ***Zheng Zhong***[1], flushed face, yellow sclera, incessant laughing, hot palms, spasms of the arms and elbows, swelling of the axillary fossa, distention, and fullness of the chest and hypochondria region.

Summary of Channel Pathology

Dominates Disorders Of	Vessels
Channel Disorder	• Channel obstruction: pain and stiffness of the neck[2], spasm of the hands and feet, swelling of the axillary fossa, inability to extend and flex the elbow, spasm of the forearm, hot palms, fullness and stuffiness of the chest and hypochondriac area. • Yellow sclera, aphasia, redness of the face.
Organ Disorder	• Heart and vessels: palpitations, Zheng Zhong, cardiac pain, restlessness, stuffiness in the chest, high lipid levels. • Mental and Emotional: delirium, syncope, incessant laughing, depression, anxiety, manic-depression.

The Clinical Applications

The points of the Pericardium Channel are mainly applied to the disorders of the chest, heart, and lung. They are also used for disorders of the stomach, and for emotional and mental disorders.

Category	Examples of Symptoms and Signs	Key points order of importance	Point combinations utilizing points from other channels.
Heart and Vessel disorders	• Palpitations, Zheng Zhong, cardiac pain, restlessness, stuffiness of the chest. • Coronary disease, high lipid levels, arteriosclerosis.	Pc 6, 4, 7 Pc 6, 5, 3	Ht 7, Ren 17, UB 15, Ki 4 St 40, Ren 17, Ht 7, Lu 9, UB 15, UB 17
Chest and Lung Disorders	• Stiffness and restricted sensation in the chest, cough, asthma, breathing difficulties.	Pc 6, 5, 4, 3	Ren 17, Lu 7, UB 13, St 40

---

[1] Zheng Zhong refers to an extreme case of palpitation as if a person were frightened or startled.

[2] The Pericardium Divergent Channel goes to the neck and connects with the mastoid process.

The Clinical Applications (continued)

Category	Examples of Symptoms and Signs	Key points order of importance	Point combinations utilizing points from other channels.
Mental and Emotional disorders	• Delirium, incessant laughing, restlessness, manic-depression, syncope, depression, anxiety.	Pc 7, 5, 6, 8, 9	Selection from 13 Ghost Points, Ht 7, Ki 4, Lu 7
Stomach disorders	• Stomach pain, distention in the epigastrium, hiccups, nausea and vomiting, cholera, food poisoning.	Pc 3, 6	St 36, St 40, Sp 4, UB 17, UB 40
Channel disorders	• Swelling of the axillary fossa, pain and spasm of the arm and elbow, hot palms, spasm of the hands and feet.	Pc 3, 7, 6, 8	Ht 1, SJ 5, LI 11,
	• Aphasia, redness of the face, yellow sclera.	Pc 7, 5, 6	Ht 5, SI 4, Du 15, Ren 23
	• Stiffness of the neck and nape, pain in the chest and hypochondriac region.	Pc 6, 4	Ht 4, SJ 5, SI 3, GB 39

The Pericardium Divergent Channel

Pathway

The Divergent Channel separates from the Pericardium Regular Channel at the level of three cun below the axillary fossa. It then enters the chest, and successively connects with each of the Three Jiaos. It then goes upward, passes through the throat, emerges at retroauricular area (mastoid process), where it converges with the San Jiao Regular Channel.

SJ ONLY DIVERGENT THAT DOESN'T ARISE FROM KNEE OR ELBOW !!!

Separates from	3 cun below the axillary fossa
Enters at the body cavity at	Chest
Connects with	Upper, middle, lower Jiao, and throat
Emerges at	Mastoid process
Converges with the San Jiao Regular Channel at	Mastoid process

Clinical Applications

The Divergent Channel reinforces the relationship between the Pericardium and San Jiao, supporting the selection of Pericardium Channel points for treating disorders of the San Jiao, and vice versa. The Pericardium Divergent Channel goes up the neck and converges with the San Jiao Regular Channel at the mastoid process, explaining the application of Pericardium Channel points for neck pain. Pc 6[1] is often used for stiffness and pain of the neck and nape, in combination with SJ 5, SJ 4, and GB 12. It is also effective for pain of the mastoid process area due to ear disorders, toothache, and Bell's Palsy.

The Divergent Channel also distributes on the side of the chest, breast, and hypochondriac region. Clinically, Pc 5 and Pc 6 are often used for disorders in those areas. Due to the connection of the Pericardium Divergent Channel with the throat, Plum Pit Qi Syndrome can be treated by Pc 5 in combination with St 40, Ht 5 and Ren 22. This combination of points can also be used for chronic throat disorders.

---

[1] Clinically, this point is needled on the ulnar side of the tendon of m. palmaris longus.

The Pericardium Tendinomuscular Channel

- Starts from: Palmar aspect of the middle finger.
- Ends at: Diaphragm.
- Qi accumulates at: Medial aspect of the elbow, below the axillary fossa, diaphragm.

Pathway

From the middle finger, the Pericardium Tendinomuscular Channel follows the Regular Channel to the medial aspect of the elbow where it **knots**, then to the area below the axillary fossa where it **knots** again. It then spreads out on sides of the chest and hypochondriac region. A branch enters the chest from the axillary fossa, distributes internally in the chest and **knots** at the diaphragm.

Pathology

1. Stiffness, pulling, spasm, pain along the course of the tendinomuscular channel.
2. Chest pain, stuffiness in the chest.
3. *Xi Fen* Syndrome. This is one of the five *Ji* syndromes (Accumulating diseases). Xi Fen Syndrome is due to stagnation of Lung Qi with accumulation of phlegm and heat. Symptoms include a mass below the right hypochondriac region (which looks like a cup with a cover on it) which may be a tumor, lung abscess, tuberculosis, or pleurisy. There may also be chest and back pain, hemoptysis, chills and fever, cough, vomiting, harsh breathing, and difficult and painful breathing.

Clinical Applications

The main application of the Pericardium Tendinomuscular Channel is pain, spasm, pulling sensation, and difficulty of movement along the medial aspect of the arm and elbow, and swelling and pain of the axillary fossa and breast.

This Tendinomuscular Channel is unusual in that it enters, and internally distributes in the chest. This explain its application to disorders of the Lung, such as Xi Fen. It is also used for muscular injury of the chest and hypochondriac region, and for costal chondritis. Pc 6 and Pc 5 are often used in combination with Ren 17, SJ 3, and St 40. It also directly connects with the diaphragm, indicating its application for hiccups, and pain and distention of the epigastrium. Pc 6 is used in combination with UB 17 and Du 9.

The Luo Collateral of Pericardium Channel

Luo point: Pc 6
Distribution: After separating from the Pericardium Regular Channel, the Luo Collateral continues with the Regular Channel to the chest, where it connects with the Pericardium and Heart system.
Connection: Pericardium, Heart system
Note: This channel is unusual in that there is no mention of connecting to its paired (San Jiao Channel).

Pathology

Excess: Cardiac pain, angina pectoris, chest pain.
Deficiency: Restlessness, irritability.

Clinical Applications

Heart disorders
Pc 6 is very effective for treating the disorders of the heart, such as cardiac pain, angina pectoris, arrhythmia, prolapse or stenosis of the mitral and tricuspid valves, tachycardia, or bradycardia. Points used in combination with Pc 6 are Pc 4, Ht 7, UB 15, Ren 17, and Ren 4.

Mental or Emotional disorders
The Luo Collateral is effective for restlessness and irritability due to excess or deficiency heat in the heart. It can also be used for depression, nervousness, and anxiety, and has the effect of lifting the spirit. Points used in combination with Pc 6 are Ht 7, Pc 7, Lv 3, SJ 3, and Du 20.

Channel disorders
Pain, spasm, and muscular tension of the arm, and numbness and tingling of the hands, such as occurs in carpal tunnel syndrome can also be treated with the Luo Collateral. Points used in combination with Pc 6 are SJ 5, Lu 7, Pc 7, and LI 4.

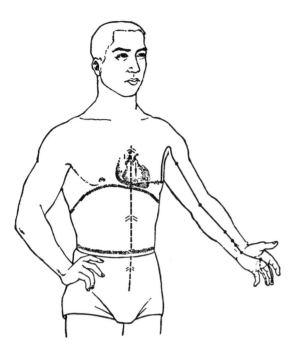

Pericardium Regular Channel

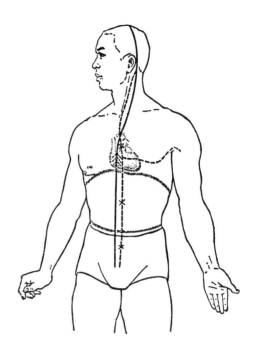

Pericardium Divergent Channel (---)
Sanjiao Divergent Channel (—)

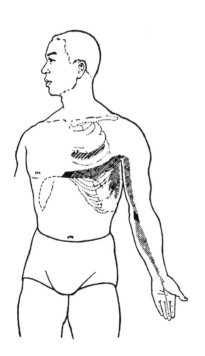

Pericardium Tendinomuscular
Channel

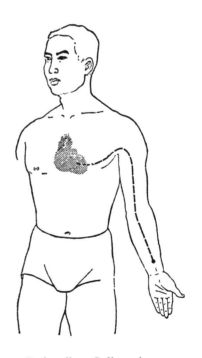

Pericardium Collateral

The Pericardium Channel of Hand-Jueyin

手 厥 陰 心 包 經 系 統 分 布 圖

10. The San Jiao Channel of Hand - Shao Yang

手 少 陽 三 焦 經

Key Points

- The San Jiao Channel starts at the ulnar side of the ring finger (SJ 1).
- The channel ends at the outer canthus (GB 1) where it connects with the Gall Bladder Channel.
- It distributes mainly on the lateromedial aspect of the upper extremities, shoulder, neck, retroauricular area and ear, cheek, and outer canthus.
- It connects with the San Jiao and pericardium.
- There are 23 points altogether.

The Pathway of the San Jiao Regular Channel

External Pathway

The San Jiao Regular Channel starts at the ulnar side of the ring finger (SJ 1), then goes toward the between the fourth and fifth metacarpals to the center of the wrist. From there, it continues up the center of the lateral aspect of the arm to the olecranon, then to the shoulder, just posterior to the clavicular-acromial joint. It then goes to and upper back (intersects SI 12 and Du 14). From Du 14, it goes to the top of the shoulder (intersects GB 21), and enters the body cavity at the supraclavicular fossa.

A branch emerges from the supraclavicular fossa. It runs on the lateral aspect of the neck, then curves around the ear on its path to the temporal region (intersects GB 6 and GB 4), then downward to the cheek (intersects SI 18), and further down to the mandible. From there, it goes up to the area below the infra orbital ridge (near St 1).

Another branch separates from behind the ear, enters the ear, then comes out again in front of it (intersects SI 19 and GB 3). It then goes to the lateral aspect of the eyebrow (SJ 23), where it links with the outer canthus (intersects GB 1) and connects with the Gall Bladder Regular Channel.

Internal Pathway

From the supraclavicular fossa, it distributes into the chest, (intersects Ren 17) and connects with the pericardium. From there, it goes down through the diaphragm to the abdomen and successively connects with the Upper, Middle, and Lower Jiaos. According to Chapter 4, "Pathogenic Qi and Zang Fu," of the Nei Jing Ling Shu (Spiritual Axis), there is a branch from the large intestine organ which descends to UB 39, the Lower He (Sea) point of the San Jiao Channel.

The Associated Organs and Points

Pertains to	Connects with	Associated With	Intersecting Points
San Jiao	Pericardium	Ear, eye, outer canthus	SI 12, Du 14, GB 21, Ren 17, GB 6, 4, SI 18, SI 19, GB 3, GB 1

Physiology

The San Jiao Channel has the following functions:

1. *Dominate the Qi of the whole body.* The San Jiao Channel is responsible for regulating and transporting Qi to the entire body. If Qi is disordered (including stagnation, excess or deficiency), it may implicate a dysfunction of the San Jiao Channel. Although the Qi stagnation may originate in any

other organ or channel (e.g., Heart, Lung, or Liver), the San Jiao Channel can have a direct influence on the Qi of the whole body. Furthermore, developments of Qi stagnation, such as stagnation of Blood and Body Fluids, which form nodules, tumors, masses, or swellings, may also indicate a disorder of the San Jiao Channel.

2. *Distribute Qi to the head and face and regulate the Qi on the sides of the body.* Symptoms such as migraine headache, ear ache, tinnitus, deafness, conjunctivitis, swollen and painful throat, hypochondriac pain, sciatica, and pain along the channel distribution may implicate a disorder of the San Jiao Channel.

3. *Regulate the body fluids circulation.* San Jiao is a water passage. This channel has a general function to regulate the upper, middle and lower source of water. It includes the function of the Lung, Spleen and Kidney. Water disorders of all kinds, such as edema, abnormal urination, dryness, and abnormal discharge may implicate a disorder of the San Jiao Channel.

4. *Treatment of Shao Yang Syndrome.* Symptoms and signs include chill and fever alternately, bitter taste in the mouth, discomfort in the chest and hypochondriac region, and poor appetite. Clinically, this syndrome can be seen in a wide range of biomedically defined conditions such as AIDS, chronic fatigue syndrome, non-specific low grade fever, fibromyalgia, and other disorders where there is latent heat.

5. *Regulate the lymphatic and endocrine systems.* Shao Yang Channel is distributed on the sides of the body which is also where many of the lymph glands are distributed. This includes the glands of the neck, axillary area, groin, chest, and sternum. In addition, the function of the endocrine system, such as the thyroid, parathyroid, pancreas, and adrenal glands are also regulated by the San Jiao Channel. Disorders such as lymphadenitis, lymphoma, hyperthyroidism and hypothyroidism, adrenocortical insufficiency, and diabetes may indicate a disorder of the San Jiao Channel.

6. *Regulate the function of the Upper, Middle, and Lower Jiaos.* The San Jiao Channel can be applied to the disorders of the Heart and Lung, Stomach and Spleen, Liver, Kidney, and the Intestines.

Pathology

Channel Pathology from the Nei Jing

The San Jiao Channel dominates the disorders of Qi. If the San Jiao Channel is disordered, there will be symptoms of deafness, blocked feeling in the ear, swollen throat, sweating, and pain of the outer canthus, cheek, and retroauricular area. There may also be pain or impaired movement along the channel distribution, including the shoulder, arm, elbow, wrist, and ring finger.

Summary of Channel Pathology

Dominates Disorders of	Qi (stagnation, excess, deficiency)
Channel Disorder	• <u>Shao Yang Syndrome</u>: chills and fever alternately, chest and hypochondriac pain, poor appetite, bitter taste in the mouth. • <u>Head, face, and sense organs</u>: migraine headache, ear pain, deafness, blocked feeling in the ear, redness and pain of the eyes, painful outer canthus, cheek and face pain, including TMJ Syndrome, toothache, mumps, swollen glands, painful throat, mandible, and retroauricular areas • <u>Channel obstruction</u>: pain and difficult lateral flexion of the neck, pain along the channel.

Organ Disorder	• **Fluid disorders**: edema, puffiness, enuresis, retention of urine, frequent urination. • **Upper Jiao**: chest pain, cough, palpitations. • **Middle Jiao**: epigastric pain, vomiting, nausea. • **Lower Jiao**: abdominal distention, fullness, constipation, diarrhea • **Lymphatic and endocrine system**: swollen glands, hypothyroidism, hyperthyroidism, diabetes. • Tumors, masses, fibroid cysts, high lipids.

The Clinical Applications

The San Jiao Channel, as is the case with the other the Yang channels of the hand, is primarily used for channel disorders. Nei Jing does not strongly emphasize its application for organ disorders. Clinically, the San Jiao Lower He (Sea) point is used for disorders of its related organs.

Category	Examples of Symptoms and Signs	Key points in order of importance	Combinations with points from other channels.
Qi disorders	• **Excess**: Distention and pain of all the organs and channels. • **Deficiency**: General lassitude, shortness of breath, fatigue, spontaneous sweating. • **Emotional disturbances**: depression, worry, low spirits, indifference.	SJ 5, 3, 7 SJ 4, 3 SJ 3, 5,16	Lv 3, LI 4 St 36, Ren 12, Ren 6, UB 43, UB 23 Du 20, Lv 3, Ki 4, Ren 6
Stagnation of Qi, Blood and Phlegm	• **Masses and tumors, nodules**: uterine fibroids, ovarian cysts, fibrocystic mastitis, abdominal masses, hernia. • High lipids, arteriosclerosis • Obesity	SJ 4, 5, 6 SJ 4, 5, 6, 12 SJ 5, 6	Ren 12, Ren 17, St 40, Lv 3, LI 4, UB 39 St 40, Sp 9, 6, UB 22, Pc 6, Pc 5 St 40, Sp 9, Lu 7, Ren 9, St 34, Sp 4
Disorders of head, face and sense organs	• Migraine headache • Otitis media, tinnitus, deafness, blocked feeling in the ear. • Redness, swelling, pain of the eyes, painful outer canthus. • Toothache, TMJ Syndrome, mumps. • Laryngitis, pharyngitis	SJ 5, 6, 3, 23 SJ 2, 3, 5, 7, 21 SJ 2, 1, 3, 23 SJ 17, 5, 7 SJ 2, 3, 5	GB 41, GB 26, GB 20 GB 41, GB 42, GB 40, Ki 6 Lv 2, GB 37, LI 4, GB 1 LI 4, LI 7, GB 41, St 44 LI 4, LI 3, Lu 7, Ki 6

The Clinical Applications (continued)

Category	Examples of Symptoms and Signs	Key points in order of importance	Point combinations utilizing points from other channels.
Shao Yang Syndrome	• Chills and fever alternately, bitter taste in the mouth, discomfort in the chest and hypochondriac region, poor appetite, et al.	SJ 5, 3, 14	GB 41, GB 34, LI 11, GB 20
	• Latent heat disorders: AIDS, chronic fatigue syndrome, non-specific low grade fever, fibromyalgia.	SJ 5, 4, 10, 3, 6	GB 41, GB 40, GB 20, Du 14, SI 3, St 36, UB 43, UB 52
Channel Disorders	• Pain, distention, muscle spasm or impaired movement of the lateral aspect of the extremities, elbow, shoulder, head and sides of the body, sciatica.	SJ 5, 3, 8, 14, 10	LI 4, LI 15, LI 11, GB 34
	• Neck sprain, stiffness, pain and difficult lateral flexion of the neck.	SJ 3, 5, 2, 7	SI 3, Luozheng, GB 39, UB 10, GB 20, UB 60
Body Fluids Disorders	• Edema, puffiness, enuresis, retention of urine, frequent urination	SJ 9, 6, 5, 4	UB 39, UB 22, UB 23, Sp 9, Ren 3, Ren 9, Lu 7, Ki 7
Disorders of the lymphatic system	• Inflammation of the lymph glands, including swollen glands of the neck, axillary fossa, and groin, lymphoma	SJ 3, 5, 17	GB 41, UB 62, LI 4, Ht 3
	• Immunodeficiency	SJ 4, 5	St 36, Du 14, UB 11, UB 13
	• Auto-immune disease, e.g., lupus, Crone's disease, multiple sclerosis	SJ 4, 5, 6	Ren 12, St 36, Sp 21, Lv 8, UB 11
Disorders of the endocrine system	• Hyperthyroidism, hypothyroidism, goiter	SJ 10, 13, 5	LI 4, LI 11, St 40, Pc 6, Ki 3
	• Diabetes, adrenocortical insufficiency	SJ 4, 5	Ren 12, St 36, Weiguanshiashu, Ki 6
	• Male and female reproductive function disorders, e.g., irregular menstruation, amenorrhea, spermatorrhea	SJ 4, 5, 3	Ren 12, Sp 6, UB 11, St 37, 39
Three Jiao disorders	• Upper Jiao: chest pain, cough, palpitations	SJ 5, 3	Ren 17, Lu 7, Pc 6
	• Middle Jiao: epigastric pain, vomiting, nausea	SJ 5, 4	Ren 12, Pc 6, St 36, Sp 4
	• Lower Jiao: abdominal distention, fullness, constipation, diarrhea, reproductive disorders	SJ 4, 5	St 37, St 39, Sp 6, Ki 6, Ren 12, UB 39

The San Jiao Divergent Channel

Pathway

The San Jiao Divergent Channel starts from the vertex (Du 20 area). It goes downward to the supraclavicular fossa, where it enters the body cavity, then connects successively with the Three Jiaos and disperses in the chest. This Divergent Channel is a special case in that: a) it starts from the vertex rather than separating from its Regular Channel on the arm, and b) the San Jiao Regular Channel has no distribution to the vertex, the Divergent Channel's origin. The connection to the vertex is explained by the theory of other channels:

- The Qi of both the Shao Yang Channel of the Hand and Foot communicate. The Hand Shao Yang connects to the vertex through the Foot Shao Yang Tendinomuscular Channel, which goes to the vertex.
- The Three Jiaos are related to the Ren and Liver Channels. Ren Channel connects with the Du Channel which reaches the vertex. The Liver Channel has a direct connection with the vertex.
- The San Jiao Regular Channel's closest point to the vertex is SJ 20, which intersects both the Gall Bladder and Urinary Bladder Channels. The Urinary Bladder Channel has a branch to the vertex.

Summary

Separates at	Vertex Du 20
Enters the body cavity at	Supraclavicular fossa
Connects with	Three Jiaos, chest
Emerges from the body cavity	None
Converges with San Jiao Regular Channel at	None

Clinical Applications

The San Jiao Divergent Channel reinforces the relationship between the Upper, Middle, and Lower Jiaos. This gives a further indication that the San Jiao Channel can be used for disorders of those areas, and their related organs.

Because of the Divergent Channel's connection to the vertex, San Jiao Channel points can be used for headache, not only on the sides, but also on the top of the head. It can also be used for dizziness and vertigo. Points often used are SJ 3 and SJ 5, in combination with Lv 3, Lv 2, GB 41, and Du 20.

San Jiao points can also be used for raising the Yang Qi and lifting the spirit. San Jiao points are useful for prolapse of the organs, light headedness, low spirits, and depression. Points often used are SJ 3 and SJ 4, in combination with Du 20, Ren 6, St 36, Sp 3, and Ki 3.

The San Jiao Divergent Channel also distributes Qi in the chest, reinforcing the use of this channel's points for treating chest disorders, such as chest stiffness and pain, cough, asthma, dyspnea, suffocating sensation, anxiety, and palpitations. Points often used are SJ 3 and SJ 5, in combination with Ren 17, Pc 6, SI 11, Lu 7, and St 40.

The San Jiao Tendinomuscular Channel

- Starts from: Ulnar side of the ring finger (SJ 1).
- Ends at: Temporofrontal area.
- Qi accumulates at: Back side of the wrist, olecranon, root of the tongue, temporofrontal area.

Pathway

The San Jiao Tendinomuscular Channel starts from the ring finger and goes to the lateral aspect of the wrist **(knots)**. It then travels up the forearm to the olecranon **(knots)**, upward along the lateral aspect of the upper arm, and over the shoulder to the neck. It joins the Small Intestine Tendinomuscular Channel at the neck. A branch from below the mandible goes to and connects with the root of the tongue **(knots)**. Another branch travels upward in front of the ear to the outer canthus, then across the temple and reaches the temporofrontal area **(knots)**. The three Yang Tendinomuscular Channels of the Hand all knot at the temporofrontal area (around St 8).

Pathology
1. Stiffness, swelling, pulling sensation along the course of the Tendinomuscular channel,
2. Curling or contracting of the tongue.

Clinical Applications
The primary application of the San Jiao Tendinomuscular Channel is for pain, stiffness, spasm, and pulling sensation along the channel distribution. This includes the sides of the head, body, and lateral aspect of the upper and lower extremities, such as Bi Syndrome, trauma, and muscular sprain.

San Jiao Channel points are also used for muscle tension and spasm due to nervous tension, emotional disturbance, or long term mental stress, especially of the neck and shoulders, hip, chest, abdomen, and knee joint. Points often used are SJ 5, SJ 6, and SJ 8, in combination with GB 34, GB 41, and Lv 3.

Because of its connection with the tongue, San Jiao Channel points are effective for tongue stiffness and speech disorders, due to curling and contraction of the tongue. This conditions is often caused by Wind Stroke. Points such as SJ 3, SJ 5, SJ 6 are used in combination with Ht 5, Lv 3, St 40, Ren 23 and Du 15.

The Luo Collateral of San Jiao Channel

Luo point:	SJ 5
Distribution:	After separating from the main channel, it follows the arm to the lateral side of the shoulder, then to the front of the chest, and communicates with the Pericardium Channel in the chest.
Connection:	Elbow, chest, Pericardium Channel.

Pathology
Excess: Spasm of the elbow joint.
Deficiency: Flaccid muscles of the arm, difficulty flexing the elbow joint.

Clinical Applications
SJ 5 covers a wide range of applications because it is not only the Luo (Connecting) point but also the Confluent point of the Yang Wei Channel. Below is a summary of its Luo (Connecting) applications.

Channel disorders
The Luo Collateral can be used for pain, spasm, and impaired movement of the elbow, wrist and arm, such as Bi Syndrome, carpal tunnel syndrome, and tennis elbow. It is also used for cervical spondylosis and nerve impairment of the forearm. Points used in combination with SJ 5 are: SJ 8, SJ 14, SJ 4, GB 34, and Lv 3.

Pain of the lateral side of the body can be treated with SJ 5, including the hip, lateral side of the lumbar area, and lower extremities, such as sciatica. Points used in combination with SJ 5 are: GB 31, GB 34, GB 26, UB 31, and Lv 3.

SJ 5 is the point which has the most influence on the Qi of the head. It can therefore be used for pain in the vertex, and temporal areas. Points used in combination with SJ 5 are GB 41, Ren 17, Ren 12, Lv 3, and Pc 6.

Organ disorders

SJ 5 can be used for disorders of the chest, heart, stomach, and Lower Jiao, such as stuffiness of the chest, breathing difficulties, palpitations, stomach pain and distention, belching, and lower abdominal pain. It is also effective for Damp Heat in the lower Jiao, which results in such symptoms as urinary dysfunction, abnormal bowel movements, and leukorrhea. Disorders of liver and gall bladder may also be treated.

Shao Yang Syndrome[1]

---

[1] For a more detailed discussion of Shao Yang Syndrome refer to the section on Yang Wei Channel.

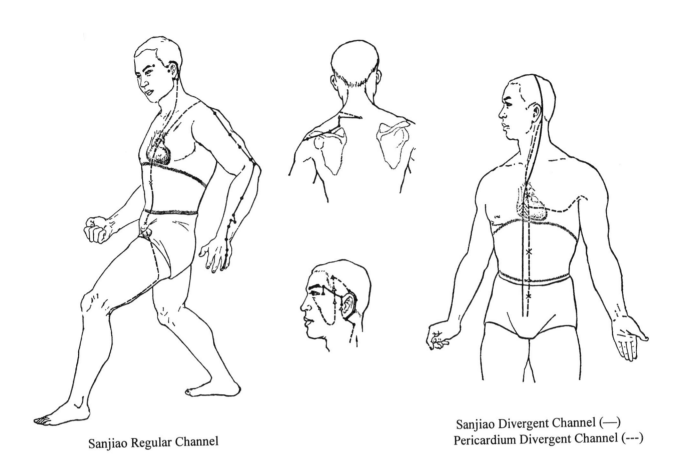

Sanjiao Regular Channel

Sanjiao Divergent Channel (——)
Pericardium Divergent Channel (---)

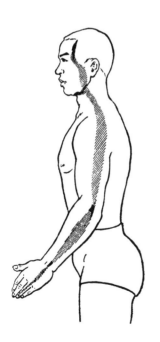

Sanjiao Tendinomuscular
Channel

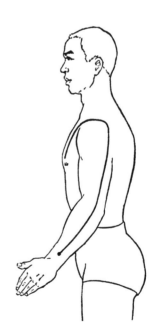

Sanjiao Collateral

The Sanjiao Channel of Hand-Shaoyang
手 少 陽 三 焦 經 系 統 分 布 圖

11. The Gall Bladder Channel of Foot - Shao Yang
足 少 陽 膽 經

Key Points
- The Gall Bladder Channel starts at the outer canthus (GB 1).
- The channel ends at the lateral aspect of the big toe (Lv 1).
- It distributes mainly on the lateral aspect of the body, including the head, eye, ear, neck, chest, abdomen, groin, hip, and lower extremities.
- It connects with the liver and gall bladder.
- There are 44 points altogether.

The Pathway of the Regular Channel

External Pathway
The Gall Bladder Regular Channel starts from the outer canthus, then traverses the lateral aspect of the head three times. From the outer canthus, it goes to the area in front of the ear (intersects SJ 22), then to the temporofrontal region (intersects St 8). It continues to the area above the ear (intersects SJ 20). It then curves around the ear to the mastoid process (intersects SI 17). From the mastoid process it goes to the forehead to the area directly over the eyebrow. From there, it travels again along the side of the head until it reaches lateral aspect of the neck (GB 20 area). From the neck it travels down to the shoulder, anterior to the San Jiao Channel, crosses it, (intersects Du 14), returns to the shoulder (intersects SI 12), and comes to the supraclavicular fossa.

A branch arises from the retroauricular area (intersects SJ 17). It then enters the ear from behind and comes out in front of it (intersects SI 19 and St 7). This branch ends at the outer canthus. Another branch starts at the outer canthus, goes down the cheek (intersects St 5), travels back up to meet the main portion of the channel, then to the infraorbital area. From there, it goes down to the cheek again (intersects St 6), then to the neck, where it meets the main pathway at the supraclavicular fossa.

The external pathway continues from the supraclavicular fossa to the area below the axillary fossa, to the lateral side of the chest (intersects Pc 1), hypochondriac region (intersects Lv 13), and lateral side of the abdomen. It goes further down to the hip and sacrum (intersects UB 31 and UB 34). It then travels along the lateral aspect of the lower extremities, passes through the external malleolus, to the foot, then between the 4th and 5th metatarsals. It ends at the lateral aspect of the fourth toe (GB 44). A branch from GB 41 goes to the lateral side of the big toe where it connects with the Liver Channel (intersects Lv 1).

Internal Pathway
The internal pathway enters the chest from the supraclavicular fossa, and passes through the diaphragm. It then pertains to the gall bladder and connects with the liver. After distributing in the hypochondriac region, and the lateral side of the abdomen, it emerges at the inguinal groove[1]. From there it goes along pubic region to the hip joint, joining the external pathway at the hip (GB 30).

---

[1] This area is called *Qi Jie*, meaning "Qi Street".

The Associated Organs and Points

Pertains to	Connects with	Associated With	Intersecting Points
Gall bladder	Liver	Heart, eye, ear	SJ 22, St 8, SJ 20, SI 17, Du 14, SI 12, SJ 17, SI 19, St 7, St 5, St 6, PC 1, Lv 13, UB 31, St 34, Lv 1

Physiology

The Gall Bladder Channel has the following functions:
1. *Regulate the Qi on the sides of the body, including the head, sense organs, trunk, and extremities.* Symptoms such as ear ache, tinnitus, conjunctivitis, migraine headache, hypochondriac pain, sciatica, and pain along the channel distribution, may suggest a disorder of the Gall Bladder Channel.
2. *Influence the bones and joints.* Since the Gall Bladder Channel's distribution on the sides of the body, it passes through many of the joints. Gall Bladder Channel points are especially good for all joint and bone disorders, such as Bi Syndrome, arthritis, osteoporosis, spondylitis, tendinitis, fibromyalgia, injury, and atony of the ligaments.
3. *Regulate the Qi in the Shao Yang Channel.* Shao Yang Syndrome, with symptoms such as alternating chills and fever, hypochondriac pain, poor appetite, and bitter taste in the mouth, may be treated with the Gall Bladder Channel.
4. *Regulate the function of the Gall Bladder and harmonize the relationship between the liver and gall bladder.* The entire digestive process, especially the secretion of bile and digestive enzymes, can be regulated by the Gall Bladder and Liver Channels. Symptoms such as pain and distention in the hypochondriac and epigastric regions, poor appetite, bitter taste in the mouth, and abnormal bowel movements, may implicate a disorder of the Gall Bladder Channel.
5. *Regulate the lymphatic system and strengthen the immunity.* The Gall Bladder and San Jiao Channels share these functions. Inflammation of the lymph glands of the neck, axillary fossa, and groin, low immunity, or autoimmune diseases can be treated by the Gall Bladder Channel.
6. *Regulate the emotions and promote mental balance.* If the Qi in the Gall Bladder Channel is normal, a person will have good judgment and be able to make prompt decisions. They will not become unreasonably angry. Abnormal emotions such as depression, mood swings, low self esteem, low spirits, poor judgment, and difficulty making decisions, may implicate a disorder of the Gall Bladder Channel.

Pathology

Channel Pathology from the Nei Jing

The Gall Bladder Channel dominates the disorders of the bones. If the channel is disordered, there may be pain of the bones and joints of the whole body. There may also be *Yang Jue Syndrome (Abnormality of Yang Qi)*, with symptoms such as bitter taste in the mouth, deep sighing, pain of the heart and hypochondriac region, difficulty rotating the body, dull and dusty facial complexion, lusterless and dry skin, and hot sensation on the lateral dorsum of the foot. Other symptoms of the Gall Bladder Channel include headache, pain of the mandible and outer canthus, pain and swelling of the supraclavicular fossa, swollen cervical and axillary lymph glands, alternating fever and chills, sweats, malaria, and pain of the chest, abdomen, hip, knee, leg (fibula), external malleolus, and fourth toe.

Summary of Channel Pathology

Dominates Disorders Of	Bones
Channel Disorder	• <u>Head, face and sense organs</u>: headache, pain in the eyes, side of cheek, ear, and mandible, deafness, tinnitus. • <u>Shao Yang Syndrome</u>: alternating chills and fever, bitter taste in the mouth, hypochondriac pain and distention, malaria. • <u>Channel obstruction</u>: pain and swelling of the neck and glands, swollen axillary fossa, pain, spasm and pulling sensation along the sides of the body, including the hip, leg, knee, fibula, ankle, and foot.
Organ Disorder	• <u>Gall bladder and liver</u>: hypochondriac pain, vomiting, nausea, belching, bitter taste in the mouth, poor appetite, abnormal bowel movements, dusty and dark complexion. • <u>Urogenital</u>: swelling and pain of the scrotum, hernia, leukorrhea, itching and pain of the external genitalia, difficult urination. • <u>Emotional and mental</u>: deep sighing, depression, mood swings, frequent anger, poor judgment, indecision, insomnia.

The Clinical Applications

The Gall Bladder Channel is mainly applied to the disorders on the side of the body. This includes migraine headache, swelling of the neck, cholecystitis, cholelithiasis, and hepatitis. It can also be used for disorders of the bones and joints.

Category	Examples of Symptoms and Signs	Key points in order of importance	Combinations with points from other channels
Channel disorders	<u>Channel obstruction</u>: pain, spasm and pulling sensation on the sides of the body, including the neck, trunk, hip, leg, external malleolus, and foot.	GB 34, 41, 31, 30	SJ 5, SJ 14, Lv 3, Sp 9
	<u>Bones and joints</u>: arthritis, osteoporosis, spondylitis, tendinitis, fibromyalgia, injury and atony of the ligaments	GB 34, 39, 30, 40	UB 11, Du 14, Lv 8, UB 65, Sp 21, SI 3
Head, face and sense organ disorders	<u>Ear</u>: Ear ache, tinnitus, deafness	GB 41, 42, 43, 40	SJ 5, SJ 2, SJ 3, SJ 17
	<u>Eye</u>: Conjunctivitis, redness of the outer canthus, retinitis, glaucoma, optic nerve atrophy	GB 37, 43, 1, 20	Lv 3, LI 11, Ki 6, SI 6
	<u>Head and face</u>: Migraine headache, TMJ syndrome, swelling of the mandible, mumps, facial pain, toothache	GB 41, 20, 34, 26	SJ 5, SJ 3, Lu 7, SJ 17, LI 4

The Clinical Applications (continued)

Category	Examples of Symptoms and Signs	Key points in order of importance	Combinations with points from other channels
Shao Yang Syndrome	Alternating chills and fever, hypochondriac pain, bitter taste in the mouth, poor appetite, nausea, vomiting	GB 41, 38, 35	SJ 5, SJ 6, Pc 6, Lv 3
Gall Bladder and Liver disorders	Hypochondriac pain or referred pain to the back and shoulder, epigastric distention, nausea, vomiting, jaundice, bitter taste in the mouth, indigestion, loose stool or constipation, dusty and dark complexion.	GB 34, 24, 41, 37, 35	Ren 12, UB 19, Lv 3, St 36, Du 9
Lymphatic and immune system disorders	Swollen glands of the neck, axillary fossa, and groin	GB 41, 40, 30, 20, 12	SJ 5, 6, 17, LI 11, St 30, UB 40
	Immunodeficiency: chronic fatigue syndrome, AIDS	GB 40, 41	SJ 4, Du 14, Ren 6, UB 43, UB 23, St 36
	Autoimmune disease	GB 40, 41	UB 19, 22, Du 14, Lv 8, St 36
Urogenital disorders	Difficult urination, stones in the urinary tract	GB 30, 41, 26, 27	Sp 6, Sp 9, Lv 5, SJ 5
	Swelling and pain of the scrotum, herpes, epidydimitis, hernia, leukorrhea, vulvitis, vaginitis, adnexitis, pelvic inflammatory disease	GB 41, 30, 26, 28	Lv 5, Lv 3, Sp 6, UB 32
Emotional and mental disorders	Poor judgment, indecision, anger, depression, mood swings, low self esteem, low spirits	GB 41, 34, 40, 24	Lv 3, LI 4, Lv 14, Pc 6

The Gall Bladder Divergent Channel

Pathway

After separating from the Regular Channel at the great trochanter (GB 30 area), the Gall Bladder Divergent Channel curves around the hip joint, then goes to the external genitalia, where it joins the Liver Divergent Channel. From there, it follows the lateral abdomen and flank, until it enters the body cavity at the hypochondriac region. It then connects with the gall bladder, liver, and further onward to connect with the heart. It continues upward, alongside the esophagus, emerges at the mandible near the mouth. From this area, it disperses in the face and connects with the eye system, and finally converges with the Gall Bladder Regular Channel at the outer canthus.

Summary

Separates from	Great trochanter (GB 30 area)
Enters the body cavity at	Hypochondriac region
Connects with	Gall bladder, liver, heart, esophagus, eye system, external genitalia
Emerges from	Mandible
Converges with the Gall Bladder Regular Channel at	Outer canthus

Clinical Applications

The Gall Bladder Divergent Channel reinforces the relationship between the gall bladder and the liver. This supports the application of the points of the Gall Bladder Channel to treat the disorders of the Liver Channel, and vice versa.

The Divergent Channel connects with the heart and esophagus. This provides the theoretical basis for using Gall Bladder Channel points for *Gall Bladder and Heart Complex*. This complex may manifest as esophagitis, gastritis, hiatal hernia, and angina pectoris-like symptoms. Symptoms such as palpitations, insomnia, being easily awakened and frightened, chest fullness and pain, suffocating sensation in the chest, burning and distention in the epigastrium or behind the sternum, sour regurgitation, and bitter taste in the mouth, are suggestive of a Gall Bladder disorder. Points often used for this condition are GB 34, GB 41, and GB 24 in combination with Lv 3, 14, Pc 7, SJ 5, and UB 19.

The Gall Bladder Regular Channel goes to the external genitalia. This reinforces the application of Gall Bladder Channel points to treat disorders of Damp Heat accumulating in the Lower Jiao. Points often used for this condition include GB 41, GB 40, and GB 30 in combination with SJ 5, Sp 9, and Lv 5.

The Gall Bladder Divergent Channel connects directly with the eye system, reinforcing the application of the Gall Bladder Channel for eye disorders. Points often used are GB 37, GB 41, and GB 1 in combination with Lv 3, SJ 5, and LI 11.

GB 30 and GB 1 are the *separating and converging points* of the Divergent Channel. They can be used alone or in combination to treat symptoms involving the hip or the eyes. For instance, GB 1 is effective in treating sciatica and pain referring to the lower extremities. The contralateral point is most effective.

The Gall Bladder Tendinomuscular Channel

- Starts from: Lateral side of the fourth toe
- Ends at: Outer canthus
- Qi accumulates at: External malleolus, lateral aspect of the knee, quadriceps, sacrum, breast, chest, hypochondriac region, supraclavicular fossa, vertex, side of the nose, and outer canthus.

Pathway

The Gall Bladder Tendinomuscular Channel starts from the fourth toe, then goes to the external malleolus, and **knots** around GB 40. From there, it follows the fibula to the side of the knee, and **knots** at the GB 34 - St 36 area.

The main portion of the pathway travels from the knee to the lateral side of the thigh, through the hip joint, hypochondriac region, and lateral side of the chest, then to the supraclavicular fossa. Along this pathway several branches diverge.

One branch diverges on the thigh and **knots** around St 32. Another branch diverges from the hip, and goes to the sacroiliac joint, where it **knots** around UB 31, then distributes to all the sacral foramina. A third branch passes anterior to the axillary region, and connects with the breast and chest.

A third branch diverges from the supraclavicular fossa, passes anterior to the Urinary Bladder Tendinomuscular Channel, then goes to the retroauricular area, and further to the temporofrontal region. There is meets the three Yang tendinomuscular channels of the hand and the Yang Qiao Channel. The Gall Bladder Tendinomuscular Channel continues to the vertex, where it meets all other channels. Each side crosses over left to right, and right to left, then goes down to the mandible area where it bifurcates. One sub-branch goes to and **knots** beside the nose, the other goes to and **knots** at the outer canthus.

Pathology

1. Stiffness and pulling sensation of the fourth toe.

2. Spasm and pulling sensation on the lateral side of the knee.
3. Impairment of movement of the knee joint.
4. Pain, spasm and pulling sensation of the popliteal fossa, which may refer to the thigh and sacral region, and vice versa.
5. Pain and pulling sensation in the sacrum region which may refer to the hypochondriac region and vice versa.
6. Pain and spasm in the supraclavicular fossa, chest, breast, and neck.
7. Spasm of the channel on the left side, which may result in inability to open the right eye, and vice versa.
8. Paralysis of the left side of the body, resulting from injury on the right temporal region[1], and vice versa.

Clinical Applications

The primary application of the Gall Bladder Tendinomuscular Channel is treating pain, muscle spasms, joint stiffness, and pulling sensation of the sides of the body. Its distribution includes many areas not covered by the Gall Bladder Regular or Divergent Channels. This additional distribution substantially extends the clinical usage of Gall Bladder Channel points.

The Gall Bladder Tendinomuscular Channel covers the anterior, lateral, and posterior aspect of the lower extremities, especially the knee and thigh. Clinically, Gall Bladder points, such as GB 34, GB 35, and GB 33, treat not only pain on the lateral side of the knee and lower extremities, but also the anterior and posterior aspects.

The Gall Bladder Tendinomuscular Channel passes through the quadriceps and further up to the sacral area. This establishes a special connection between St 32 and UB 31. Lower back pain or sciatica, which refers to the lower extremities, can be treated with St 32 and UB 31, in combination with GB 29 or GB 30.

The Tendinomuscular Channel also distributes on the chest and breast, indicating its points may be selected for pain and spasm of these areas. Points such as GB 41, GB 40, and GB 21, in combination with SJ 6 and SJ 5, are often used. Disorders which may be treated in this manner include fibrocystic breast disorders, mastitis, pleurisy, and herpes zoster.

The Gall Bladder Tendinomuscular Channel is important for treating the sequelae of Wind Stroke, and blepharoptosis due to facial paralysis. Paralysis on one side of the body is generally treated by contralateral points. GB 34, GB 31, and GB 39, are used in combination with LI 15, LI 11, SJ 5, and St 36.

The Tendinomuscular Channel can also be applied for headache. This includes pain at the vertex, pain on the sides of the head, either of which may refer to the eyes or neck. Points often used include GB 41, GB 20, and GB 4, in combination with SJ 5, SJ 23, Lv 2, and Du 20.

Acute or chronic nose disorders, such as sinusitis, rhinitis, nasal polyps, and allergy, are often treated with Gall Bladder points. The Tendinomuscular Channel knots at the nose, establishing a connection between the Gall Bladder Channel and the nose. Points such as GB 40, GB 41, GB 35, are often used in combination with SJ 3, SJ 5, and St 36.

The Gall Bladder Luo Collateral

Luo point: GB 37
Distribution: After separating from the Gall Bladder Regular Channel at GB 37, the Luo Collateral makes a network to connect with the Liver Channel. It then goes down, distributing on the dorsum of the foot.

---

[1] Paralysis of one side of the body was explained in the Nei Jing to be due to injury of the temporal region. This includes CVA or extreme trauma to the head causing internal bleeding.

Connection: Dorsum of the foot, Liver Channel

Pathology

<u>Excess:</u>   Cold sensation of the feet.
<u>Deficiency:</u>   Weakness, flaccidity of the muscles of the foot, causing difficulty standing; paralysis of the lower extremities.

Clinical Applications

Channel disorders

The Luo Collateral can be used for pain, spasm, pulling sensation, and weakness of the lower extremities and feet. It is especially applicable to symptoms on the lateral and posterior aspects. Points used in combination with GB 37 are: Lv 3, GB 34, UB 40, and St 36.

Eye Disorders

Due to its direct connection with the Liver Channel, GB 37 has a strong effect on eye disorders of all kinds. The name of this point, *Guang Ming*, means *Brightness of the Eyes*. Points often used in combination with GB 37 are: Lv 3, LI 4, and UB 18.

Organ disorders

The Luo (Connecting) point can be used for disorders of the liver and gall bladder, such as hepatitis, cholecystitis, and cholelithiasis. It is also used for emotional symptoms, including anger, frustration, and depression. Points often used in combination with GB 37 are: Lv 3, Lv 6, GB 24, Pc 6, LI 4, and UB 18.

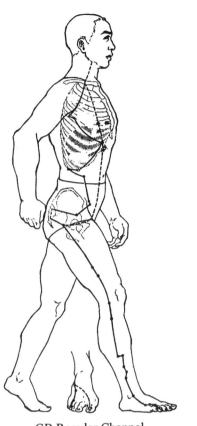

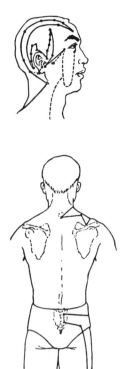

GB Regular Channel

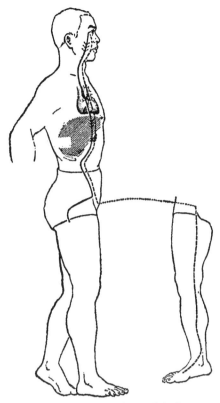

GB Divergent Channel (—)
Liver Divergent Channel (---)

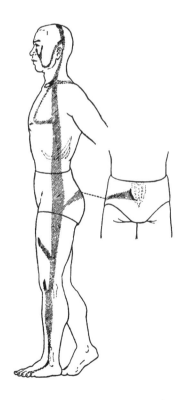

GB Tendinomuscular Channel

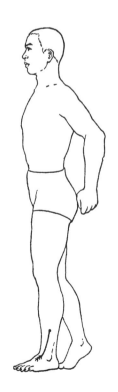

GB Collateral

The Gallbladder Channel of Foot-Shaoyang
足 少 陽 膽 經 系 統 分 布 圖

12. The Liver Channel of Foot - Jue Yin

足 厥 陰 肝 經

Key Points
- The Liver Channel starts at the lateral side of the big toe (Lv 1).
- The channel ends at the hypochondriac region (externally), vertex, and connects with the Lung Channel in the chest (internally).
- It distributes mainly on the medial aspect of the lower extremities, abdomen, chest, nasopharynx, eyes, lips, and vertex.
- It connects with liver, gall bladder, stomach, lung, and brain.
- There are 14 points altogether.

The Pathway of the Liver Regular Channel

External Pathway
The Liver Regular Channel starts on the lateral aspect of the big toe, in the hairy region. It follows the dorsum of the foot to the area anterior to the medial malleolus, then goes up the leg on the medial aspect (intersects Sp 6). At the level of 8 cun above the medial malleolus, it crosses the Spleen Channel.. From there, it goes along the medial aspect of the knee and thigh, running between the Spleen and Kidney Channels, then to the inguinal groove, 2.5 cun lateral to the Ren channel (intersects Sp 12, Sp 13). It curves around the external genitalia, traveling lateral to the Stomach Channel, and goes through the abdomen to the hypochondriac region, where it ends (Lv 14).

Internal Pathway
The internal pathway begins when it enters the abdomen at Sp 13. It passes through the lower abdomen (intersects Ren 2, Ren 3, and Ren 4), then along side the stomach, and enters the liver, its pertaining organ. It then connects with the gall bladder, penetrates the diaphragm, and distributes in the chest and hypochondriac region. It continues upward, along the posterior aspect of the trachea, to the nasopharynx, connects with the eye system, then passes through the forehead to the vertex (intersects Du 20), where it ends. A branch from the liver goes through the diaphragm to the Lung and connects with the Lung Channel in the chest, where it ends. A branch from the eye system goes down the cheek and encircles the lips.

The Associated Organs and Points

Pertains to	Connects with	Associated With	Intersecting Points
Liver	Gall bladder	External genitalia, stomach, lung, diaphragm, trachea nasopharynx, eye system, lips, brain.	Sp 6, Sp 12, Sp 13, Ren 2, Ren 3, Ren 4, Du 20

Physiology

The Liver Channel has the following functions:
1. *Promote the free flow of Qi throughout the whole body.* By doing so, it consequently smoothes the circulation of the blood and body fluids. If the Liver Qi is stagnated, there will be distention and pain on the course of the Liver Channel, which may also affect the other channels and organs. Symptoms

such as lower back pain, headache, body aches, and joint pain, may occur. The Liver Channel also has the function of purification and detoxification. In TCM, stagnation or heat in the blood, and retention of body fluids, are considered manifestations of toxic accumulations in the body and may also indicate a disorder of the Liver Channel.

2. *Regulate mental function and the emotions.* Symptoms such as nervousness, dizziness, depression, anger, and frustration may suggest a disorder of the Liver Channel.

3. *Regulate and balance the function of the internal organs.*
   a) Liver and gall bladder. The Liver Channel regulates the function of its own pertaining and connecting organs. Clinically, hepatitis, cholecystitis, cholelithiasis, cirrhosis, and hypofunction of the liver, can be treated with Liver Channel points.
   b) Spleen and stomach. The Liver Channel harmonizes the relationship between the liver, stomach and spleen. It influences the ascending and descending functions of the Spleen and Stomach Qi. It regulates the entire digestive process, including the release of bile. Symptoms such as epigastric pain, nausea, vomiting, jaundice, and diarrhea may indicate a disorder of the Liver Channel.
   c) Kidney and urinary bladder. The Liver Channel circulates around and through the external genitalia, and regulates the reproductive and urinary functions. Disorders related to menstruation, pregnancy, lactation, and vaginal discharge, may be indications of a Liver Channel disorder. This is also true for male reproductive diseases, hernia, impotence, cystitis, and retention of urine,
   d) Heart and lung. The Liver Channel passes through the chest and hypochondriac region, connects with the Lung, and regulates the circulation of Qi in the chest. Symptoms such as chest pain, stuffiness of the chest, cough with blood tinged sputum, palpitations, and insomnia, may implicate a Liver Channel disorder.

4. *Regulate the endocrine system.* The Liver Channel regulates the function of the endocrine system, including the pancreas, thyroid, adrenal, pituitary glands, and ovaries. Disorders such as diabetes, hypothyroidism, and hyperthyroidism, may be related to a disorder of the Liver Channel.

Pathology

Channel Pathology from the Nei Jing

The Liver Channel dominates the disorders of the Liver. If the Liver Channel is disordered, there will be chest fullness, nausea and vomiting after eating, diarrhea, enuresis, and retention of urine. Other symptoms of the Liver Channel include lumbar pain with difficulty in bending forward and backward, hernia[1], swelling of the lateral lower abdomen, dry throat, dusty face, and change of skin color (dusty, dark, lusterlessness, and small dark purplish veins on the face).

Seven Shan (Hernia)

There are seven types of ***Shan*** mentioned in the Nei Jing and further explained in other medical classics.

1. Hu Shan - (Fox Hernia)

This is an inguinal hernia. The name refers to the sudden nature of its onset, like the movement of a fox, which comes and goes. The scrotum enlarges when part of the small intestine drops down. It can be pushed back in place when lying down, and falls down again when standing for a long time.

2. Han Shan - (Cold Hernia)

The name refers to two conditions:
   a) Swelling, pain, coldness and hardness of the scrotum and testicles, accompanied by impotence and cold appearance.

---

[1] There are seven types of hernia mentioned in the Nei Jing, but little explanation is offered. Later generations detailed the description of these disorders. The material in this text is from those sources, i.e., Zhu Bing Yuan Hou Lun (Treatise on the Sources and Explanation of all Diseases), I Zhong Bi Du (Essential Medical Book).

b) Pain and cramps of the lower abdomen, which may refer to the umbilicus or hypochondriac region. This is often due to Yang Deficiency of the Spleen and Stomach, or Blood Deficiency during the post-partum period accompanied by external attack of Wind Cold. This condition is not a true hernia but is categorized under Han Shan.

3. Qi Shan - (Qi Hernia)

This is swelling and pain of the scrotum (often unilateral, sometime alternating), which refers to the lower back. It occurs mostly in children. The scrotum often enlarges when they are angry, cry, or scream. The scrotum will go back to a normal size after the upset emotions subside.

4. Tui Shan - (This term has several meanings)

a) *Swollen Hernia*. In men this is swelling of the scrotum without pain or itching. In women it refers to a prolapse of the uterus

b) *Abdominal Abscess Hernia*. The abscess can be located in the intestines, appendix, or fallopian tubes. This condition is often accompanied by retention of urine.

c) *Discharge Hernia*. This refers to a condition of the external genitalia, with constant discharge, which can be purulent or non-purulent, and is due to inflammation or infection.

5. Shui Shan - (Water Shan)

The name refers to two conditions:

a) Swelling, pain, and sweating of the scrotum with a yellow discharge (hydrocele of the tunica vaginalis).

b) Itching and dryness of the scrotum with discharge. This is often caused by Kidney deficiency accompanied by invasion of Wind Cold and accumulation of dampness.

6. Chong Shan - (Rushing Qi Sensation Hernia)

This condition refers to pain and distention, rushing from the lower abdomen to the chest, heart area, or even the head and face. Common symptoms are asthma, difficulty breathing, chest stuffiness, sweating, hot flashes, anxiety, and palpitations, sometimes accompanied by constipation and retention of urine.

7. Jing Shan - (Penis Hernia)

This refers to contraction and pain of the penis. There may be swelling, itching and lesions with discharge, as in syphilis, gonorrhea, and other venereal diseases. It may be accompanied by impotence or white discharge in the urine. This condition is often due to Damp Heat in the Liver Channel.

Summary of Channel Pathology

Dominates Disorders Of	Liver
Channel Disorder	• <u>Channel obstruction</u>: Spasm of hands and feet, lower back pain, headache, lumbar pain which refers to the scrotum, hernia, swelling of the lateral abdomen, spasm and tightness of the muscles and joints, and disorders along the channel distribution.
Organ Disorder	• <u>Liver Qi and Yang</u>: hypochondriac pain, fullness, distention, dizziness, blurred vision, tinnitus, dry throat, flushed face, fever, jaundice, bitter taste in the mouth. • <u>Mental and emotional</u>: nervousness, depression, mood swings, frequent anger, frustration. • <u>Stomach and spleen</u>: epigastric distention, belching, flatulence, eating disorders, nausea, vomiting, diarrhea, abdominal pain, and distention (continued on next page)

Summary of Channel Pathology (continued)

Organ Disorder (continued)	<ul><li>Urogenital: irregular menstruation, infertility, leukorrhea, itching and burning sensation of the external genitalia, impotence, spermatorrhea, epidydimitis, orchitis, enuresis, retention of urine, and yellow urination.</li><li>Lung and heart: stuffiness of chest, cough with blood tinged sputum, shallow breathing, deep sighing, palpitations, and dream-disturbed sleep.</li><li>Liver Qi and phlegm obstruction: abnormal growths including masses, nodules, fibroids and cysts, Plum Pit Qi.</li></ul>

The Clinical Applications

The points of the Liver Channel are mainly applied to the disorders of Liver Qi stagnation and its consequences, such as blood stagnation and body fluid disorders. It is also used for mental, emotional, and endocrine system disorders.

Category	Examples of Symptoms and Signs	Key points in order of importance	Combinations with points from other channels
Liver Qi Stagnation	• Stagnation of Qi in the Channels: pain and distention in the lateral abdomen, hypochondriac region, lower back pain, spasm of the hands and feet, tightness and spasm of the muscles and joints, headache (vertex, temporal, occipital areas), and symptoms along the channel distribution.	Lv 3, 2, 5, 6, 14	LI 4, UB 40, GB 41, SJ 5, Ren 17
	• Liver and Gall Bladder: pain and distention in the hypochondriac region, and chest, bitter taste in the mouth, jaundice, redness and swelling of the eye and ear, abnormal discharge of the external genitalia.	Lv 3, 14, 2, 5, 6	LI 4, Ren 12, SJ 5, GB 41, Pc 6, Ht 7, GB 34
	• Emotional and mental: depression, anger, frustration, mood swings	Lv 2, 3, 14, 4	Pc 6, LI 4, Ht 7, Sp 6, Ren 17

The Clinical Applications (continued)

Category	Examples of Symptoms and Signs	Key points in order of importance	Combinations with points from other channels
Disorders developed from Liver Qi Stagnation	• Liver Fire flaring up: headache, red face, red and painful eyes, irritability.	Lv 2, 3, 4, 14	GB 43, Taiyang, SJ 1, Sp 6
	• Liver Yang Hyperactivity: headache, dizziness, vertigo, blurring of vision, tinnitus, flushed face, irritability.	Lv 2, 3, 4, 14	LI 4, SJ 5, GB 41, Sp 6, Ki 6, Du 20
	• Blood Stagnation: stabbing pain, purple tongue, dark and dusty complexion, irregular menstruation.	Lv 3, 2, 6	LI 4, UB 40, Pc 3, Sp 10
	• Body fluid retention: edema, puffiness of the face, retention of urine, heavy sensation of the body.	Lv 3, 8, 5	SJ 6, Sp 6, Sp 9, UB 39
	• Qi and Phlegm obstruction: abnormal growths, masses, tumor, cysts, fibroids, obesity, Plum Pit Qi.	Lv 3, 4, 5, 14	St 40, Sp 10, Sp 9, Ren 6, 17, UB 22, Pc 6
Spleen and Stomach disorders	• Epigastric distention or burning, belching, nausea, vomiting, sour regurgitation, flatulence, diarrhea, constipation, eating disorders, abdominal pain, food sensitivity.	Lv 13, 3, 2, 14	Pc 6, Sp 4, St 36, GB 34, Ren 12
Urogenital disorders	• Reproductive: Irregular menstruation, dysmenorrhea, endometriosis, leukorrhea, infertility, hernia, impotence, vulvitis, genital herpes.	Lv 3, 5, 8, 12, 1	Sp 6, GB 41, UB 32, Ren 4
	• Urinary: Painful and difficult urination, retention of urine, enuresis.	Lv 5, 8, 3	Sp 9, Sp 6, Lu 7, Ki 6, Ren 3, St 28
Lung and Heart disorders	• Lung: Chest pain and stuffiness, deep sighing, shallow breathing, cough with blood tinged sputum.	Lv 4, 3, 2	Lu 7, Pc 6, LI 4, Ki 6
	• Heart: palpitations, dream-disturbed sleep, insomnia.	Lv 3, 8, 2, 14	Ht 7, Pc 6, Ren 17, Ki 4
Endocrine disorders	• Diabetes, hyperthyroidism, hypothyroidism, adrenal cortical insufficiency, pituitary disorders, hormonal imbalances	Lv 3, 8, 6	Ren 12, SJ 4, UB 22, UB 20, Weiguanxiashu, UB 23

The Liver Divergent Channel

Pathway

After separating from the Liver Regular Channel at the dorsum of the foot, the Divergent Channel follows the Regular Channel to the external genitalia, where it joins Gall Bladder Divergent Channel and follows it to its end at the outer canthus.

Separates from	Dorsum of the foot
Qi accumulates at	External genitalia
Enters body cavity at	Same as Gall Bladder Divergent
Connects with	Same as Gall Bladder Divergent (Gall bladder, liver, heart, esophagus, eye system, external genitalia)
Emerges from	Same as Gall Bladder Divergent (Mandible)
Converges with Gall Bladder Regular Channel at	Same as Gall Bladder Divergent (Outer canthus)

Clinical Applications

the Liver Divergent Channel reinforces the connection between the Liver Channel and the external genitalia, supporting the use of Liver Channel points for treatment of urogenital disorders. Lv 5 and Lv 8 are often used in combination with GB 41, SJ 5, Ren 3, St 28, and Sp 6.

The Liver and Gall Bladder Divergent Channels separate at Lv 3 and GB 30 respectively, and converge at the external genitalia. From there, they travel together, ending at GB 1. This demonstrates the relationship between Lv 3, GB 30, the external genitalia, and the eye. GB 1 can be used for treating the disorders of the hip and lower extremities, such as sciatica, injury of the foot, impaired movement of the leg, and neuropathies of the foot. Lv 3 can be used in combination with GB 30 for the disorders of the genital area, and eyes.

The Liver Tendinomuscular Channel

- Starts from: Dorsum of the big toe
- Ends at: External genitalia
- Qi accumulates at: Medial malleolus, medial aspect of the knee, external genitalia.

Pathway

The Liver Tendinomuscular Channel starts from the dorsum of the big toe, goes in front of the medial malleolus (knots), ascends along the medial aspect of the tibia, then goes to the medial aspect of the knee (knots). From the knee it goes upward on the medial aspect of the thigh, then to the external genitalia, where it connects with the many other tendinomuscular channels which go there.

Pathology
1. Stiffness, spasm, and pulling sensation of the big toe.
2. Pain of the medial malleolus.
3. Pain at the medial aspect of the knee (around Lv 7 and Lv 8).
4. Pain and muscle spasm of the medial aspect of the thigh.
5. Dysfunction of the external genitalia:
   a. Impotence caused by excessive sexual indulgence or Damp Heat.
   b. Spasm of the external genitalia caused by external or internal Damp Cold.
   c. Pain or abnormal discharge of the external genitalia caused by external or internal Heat.

Clinical Applications

The primary application of the Liver Tendinomuscular Channel is for pain, spasm, and pulling sensation along the channel distribution. This includes the big toe, the medial aspect of the lower extremities, and the lateral side of the abdomen. It is also effective for contraction of the muscles of the medial aspect of the lower extremities, and the consequent inversion of the foot which result from it.

The external genitalia is the place where the Qi of the Liver Regular, Divergent, Tendinomuscular Channels, and Luo Collateral converge. Consequently, Liver Channel points are the first choice when treating disorders of this area. Lv 1 and Lv 5 may be used to treat such symptoms as muscle spasm (or flaccidity), pain, pulling sensation, and distending sensations of the external genitalia. These symptoms are often seen in cases of hernia, prostatitis, orchitis, and impotence.

The Luo Collateral of Liver Channel

Luo point: Lv 5
Distribution: After separating from the Liver Regular Channel, the Luo Collateral connects with the Gall Bladder Channel, then follows the Regular Channel up the thigh, encircles the external genitalia, and converges at the penis.
Connection: External genitalia including the testicles, penis, and Gall Bladder Channel

Pathology
Excess: Constant erection.
Deficiency: Itching of external genitalia, (e.g., herpes, eczema, candida, vulvitis).
Rebellious Qi: Swelling and pain of testicles and scrotum, hernia.

Clinical Applications

Urogenital Disorders
Lv 5 has a strong effect on the external genitalia and has the specific function of resolving Damp Heat. It can be used for all disorders of the external genitalia, both male and female. It is also useful for difficult and painful urination, leukorrhea, eczema, candida, vulval abscess, and genital herpes. Points used in combination with Lv 5 are Lv 8, Sp 6, Ren 2, Ren 3, St 28, SJ 5, and GB 41.

Liver and Gall Bladder Disorders
Lv 5 can be used for disorders of both liver and gall bladder, such as hepatitis, cholecystitis and cholelithiasis. Points used in combination with Lv 5 are Lv 6, GB 40, Lv 14, GB 41, and GB 34.

Channel Disorders
The Luo Collateral can be used for pain and contraction on both lateral and medial aspects of the lower extremities, such as sciatica. Points used in combination with Lv 5 are GB 40, GB 34, and Pc 6.

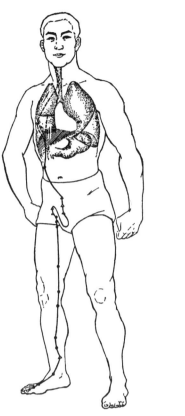

Liver Regular Channel

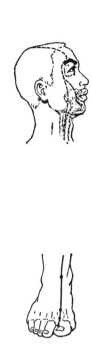

Liver Divergent Channel (---)
GB Divergent Channel (—)

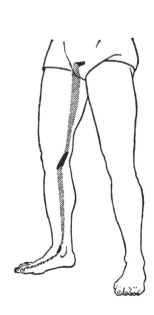

Liver Tendinomuscular
Channel

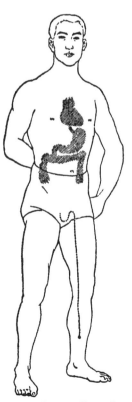

Liver Collateral

The Liver Channel of Foot-Jueyin
足厥陰肝經系統分布圖

The Eight Extraordinary Channels

The symptomology presented for the Eight Extraordinary Channels is compiled from the Nei Jing (Spiritual Axis and Plain Questions), Nan Jing (Classic of Difficulties), Qi Jing Ba Mai Kao (Research on the Eight Extraordinary Channels) and later medical commentaries.

The Du Channel

督 脉

Key Points

- *Du* means governing or dominating.
- The Du Channel governs all Yang Channels. It is the Sea of Yang Qi.
- The distribution of the Du channel is mainly on the central aspect of the back and head.
- It connects mainly with the uterus, kidney, heart, and brain.
- There are 28 point altogether.

The Pathways of the Du Channel

Du Channel has four pathways:

1. Starts at the perineum (intersects Ren 1), then follows the spinal column up to the nape area (Du 16) where a branch enters and connects with the brain. The main channel continues to the vertex, and follows the forehead to the nose, (Du 26) and ends at the frenulum of the upper lip (Du 28).
2. Starts from the uterus in women, deep inside Ren 4 for men, which is the same starting point as the Chong and Ren Channels. From there, it goes down to the external genitalia and perineum, then follows the sides of the coccyx, where it joins the Kidney and Urinary Bladder Channels (around UB 35). Together with these two other channel, the Du Channel goes to the middle of the sacrum, up to the lumbar region, enters the body cavity, and connects with the kidney.
3. Starts at the inner canthus (UB 1), then follows the course of the Urinary Bladder Channel to the vertex and enters the brain. It emerges, then goes down the nape, then follows the first line of the Urinary Bladder Channel (intersects UB 12) to the lumbar region, where it enters the body and connects with the kidney again.
4. Starts from the lower abdomen (Ren 4 area), then takes the course of the Ren Channel, and passes through the umbilicus. It continues upward through the Heart center and connects with the throat, where the Du, Ren, and Chong Channels meet. It then goes to the cheek, curves around the lips, and ends below the eye.

The Associated Organs, Areas and Points

Du Channel	
Starting and ending of each pathway	1. Perineum/Frenulum (Du 28) 2. Uterus/Spinal Column 3. Inner canthus/kidney 4. Lower abdomen (Ren 4 area)/below the eyes

Associated areas of each pathway	1. Perineum, external genitalia, anus, spinal column and spinal cord, lumbar area, back, nape, vertex, forehead, and nose. 2. Uterus, perineum, anus, coccyx, sacrum, spinal column, and kidney. 3. Eye, vertex, brain, Urinary Bladder Channel first line, and kidney 4. Center of the lower and upper abdomen, umbilicus, chest, heart center, front of the neck, cheek, lips, and eye.
Connected organs	Uterus, kidney, heart, brain
Coincides with	Urinary Bladder, Ren, and Chong Channels
Intersecting points	Ren 1, UB 12
Confluent and Paired Point	SI 3, UB 62

Physiology

The Du Channel has the following functions:
1. *Govern all the Yang Channels.* The Du Channel is called the **Sea of Yang Qi**. Its distribution is mainly on the Yang aspect of the body, all six regular Yang channels meet the Du Channel at Du 14, and the Yang Wei, Yang Qiao, and Dai Channels intersect Du Channel at Du 4, Du 16, and Du 15. This completes the convergence of all Yang Qi in the Du Channel.
2. *Provide heat (Yang Qi) to warm all the organs and channels.* Du Channel points can be used to treat the disorders of all Yang Channels, and all syndromes due to either excess or deficiency of Yang Qi.
3. *Influence the function of the brain, head, and sense organs.* The Du channel directly connects with the brain and spinal column, and is used to treat brain, mental, emotional, and nervous system disorders. It can also be used to treat disorders of the head, face, eyes, nose, mouth, and lips.
4. *Strengthen the body constitution and enhance the immunity.* The Du Channel circulates the Yang Qi to nourish the marrow and bones. It is related to the function of Kidney Yang and Jing. Symptoms such as slow growth, congenital defects, and low immunity can be treated by this channel.
5. *Regulate the function of its associated organs and channels.* The Du Channel not only regulates the function of the uterus, kidney, heart and brain, it also influences the function of all the other channels and organs because of two important connections. 1) One of its pathways coincides with the Ren Channel and the Chong Channel. The Ren Channel is the Sea of Yin Qi, and is connected to all Yin Channel. The Chong Channel is the Sea of the Twelve Channels because its pathways coincide with both the Ren and Du Channels. 2) By virtue of its connection with the Urinary Bladder Channel first line, it connects with all twelve channels through the Back Shu points.

Pathology

When the Qi of the Du Channel is disordered, there may be stiffness and pain along the spinal column, opisthotonos, manic-depression, disorders due to Wind such as Wind Stroke, epilepsy, infantile convulsions, shaking, tremors, heavy sensation of the head, dizziness, vertigo, fever, Qi rushing upward, hemorrhoids, enuresis, retention of urine, and pain along the channel distribution.

The Clinical Applications of the Du Channel

The points of the Du Channel are mainly applied to the disorders of the brain and nervous system, mental and emotional disorders. It also treats the back, head, sense organs, febrile diseases, disorders of Yang Qi and the Zang/Fu organs.

Category	Examples of Symptoms and Signs	Key points in order of importance	Combinations with points from other channels.
Disorders of Yang Qi	• Heat syndromes Excess: Febrile diseases, heat syndromes of Zang/Fu organs.	Du 14, 13	LI 11, SJ 5, LI 4, St 44, Shixuan
	Deficiency: Deficiency heat syndromes of Zang/Fu organs.	Du 14, 12, 13, 9	SI 3, Ki 7, Ht 5, UB 43, Ki 6
	• Cold syndromes Excess: Exterior and interior Cold syndromes.	Du 14, Du 9	UB 12, LI 4, Lu 7, SJ 5, St 36, Sp 6
	Deficiency: Yang Qi deficiency.	Du 4, 3	Ren 4, St 36, UB 13, UB 23, UB 21
Disorder of the brain, emotional, mental and nervous system disorders	• Dian Kuang, violent behavior, schizophrenia.	Du 1, 16, 15, 20, 26	SI 3, selection of 13 Ghost Points
	• Depression, anger, anxiety, worry, fright, fear, melancholy.	Du 20, 11, 4	Lv 3, Ht 7, Ki 4, LI 4, St 40
	• Epilepsy, Wind Stroke, convulsions, coma, syncope, opisthotonos.	Du 2, 20, 26, 16, 24	Shixuan, Jing (Well) points, SI 3, UB 62, Ki 6, Ren 15
	• Neuropathies, neuromuscular diseases, nervous tension.	Du 8, 3, 24	Lv 3, GB 34, Pc 6, Ht 7
Congenital and degenerative Disorders, Immuno-deficiency	• Slow growth, congenital defects, weakness and degeneration of the bones and joints, weak constitution	Du 4, 12, 14	UB 23, Ki 3, GB 39, UB 11
	• Chronic disease, AIDS, chronic fatigue syndrome, autoimmune disease.	Du 14, 4, 12, 9	St 36, Ki 3, UB 23, UB 43, Ren 6
Head, Face and Sense Organ Disorders	• Stiffness and rigidity of the neck, dizziness, vertigo, headache.	Du 16, 20	UB 10, SI 3, Lv 2, Lv 3, GB 20, Lu 7
	• Blurring of vision, acute or chronic eye disorders.	Du 4, 16, 23	Lv 3, GB 37, GB 20, LI 4
	• Acute or chronic sinusitis, rhinitis, obstruction of the nose, epistaxis	Du 23, 20, 12	LI 4, St 40, Lu 7, UB 7, GB 20
	• Aphasia, aphonia due to Wind Stroke, deaf mutism, swollen and painful throat.	Du 15, 16	St 40, Ht 5, LI 4
Urogenital Disorders	• Retention of urine, enuresis, hemorrhoids, prostatitis.	Du 3, 2, 4, 1	Ren 3, Ren 4, Ren 1, Sp 6, UB 34, UB 57, Lu 6
	• Infertility, irregular menstruation, impotence, premature ejaculation, oligospermia.	Du 4, 3, 2	Sp 6, Ren 4, St 36, Ki 6, UB 23, Shiqizhuixia

The Clinical Applications of the Du Channel (continued)

Category	Examples of Symptoms and Signs	Key points in order of importance	Combinations with points from other channels
Qi Rushing Up Sensation Syndrome (Chong Shan)[1]	• Flatulence, asthma, hot flashes and sweating, anxiety attack, palpitations, insomnia, acute stomach pain and distention, or hiatal hernia, constipation, retention of urine.	Du 4, 11, 9, 20	UB 11, St 37, St 39, Lv 3, Sp 4, Pc 6, Sp 6
Disorders of Internal Organs	• <u>Kidney</u>: Deficiency of Qi, Yin, Yang, and Jing.	Du 4, 3, 12, 14	UB 23, Ki 3, Ki 6, Ki 7, GB 39, Ren 4
	• <u>Heart</u>: palpitations, stuttering, arrhythmia, nightmare.	Du 11, 9, 4	Ht 7, Pc 6, UB 15, St 36, St 44, Sp 1
	• <u>Lung</u>: asthma, cough, breathing difficulties, allergy.	Du 12, 13	UB 13, UB 17, SI 11, Lu 7
	• <u>Liver</u>: hepatitis, jaundice.	Du 9, 8, 7	UB 18, Lv 3, GB 37
	• <u>Spleen, stomach, intestines</u>: indigestion, epigastric pain, diarrhea, vomiting, constipation.	Du 9, 6, 5, 4, 3	UB 20, UB 21, UB 25, UB 27, St 36, Sp 4, St 37
	• <u>Prolapse of internal organs</u>: uterus, stomach, rectum, kidney	Du 20, 2, 4, 3	Ren 4, Ren 6, Ren 12, UB 23, St 36
	• <u>Uterus</u>: see urogenital disorders		
	• <u>Brain</u>: see mental and emotional disorders		
Channel Obstruction	• Acute lower back pain	Du 26, 20	SI 3, Yaotongdian, UB 40
	• Pain, spasm of the nape, back, lower back and legs, Bi syndrome	Du 14, 16, 9, 3, local points	SI 3, UB 62, GB 34, LI 4, Lv 3, UB 40, UB 58

The Luo Collateral of Du Channel

Luo point: Du 1
Distribution: After separating from the Du Channel at tip of the coccyx (Du 1), it goes along the sides the spinal column, through the area of the Huatuojiaji points, up to the nape, and distributes in the head. At the scapula region, a branch goes to and connects with the first line of the Urinary Bladder Channel.
Connection: Anus, spinal column, nape, head, and Ren Channel.
Coincides with: Urinary Bladder Channel first line.

Pathology
<u>Excess</u>:   Rigidity and stiffness of the spinal column.
<u>Deficiency</u>:   Heavy sensation of the head, dizziness, vertigo.

---

[1] Chong Shan involves a sensation of pain and distention which rushes from the lower abdomen to the chest and heart area. It causes difficulty breathing, chest stuffiness or sweating, hot flashes, anxiety and palpitations. It can be accompanied by constipation and retention of urine.

Clinical Applications

Channel Disorders

Du 1 can be used for all the disorders of the back, spinal column, and adjacent muscles including cervical spondylosis, thoracic and lumbar arthritis, and disc herniation and degeneration. Points used in combination with Du 1 are SI 3, UB 62, Du 14, UB 11, Du 3, GB 39, and Ki 3.

Head Disorders

Du 1, being located at the end of the spine, has an effect on the top of the head. It is effective for vertigo, dizziness, and headache, which are frequently caused by Liver Yang Hyperactivity or Liver Wind with congealed Phlegm (often present in Wind Stroke). Points used in combination with Du 1 are Lv 3, Lv 2, LI 4, St 40, SJ 5, and Sp 6.

Mental and Emotional Disorders

Du 1 has a strong effect on the brain. It is used for symptoms such as epilepsy, manic-depression, and schizophrenia, and to calm the mind. It is, therefore, useful for diseases characterized by agitation or hypomania. Points used in combination with Du 1 are SI 3, UB 62, Ren 15, along with a selection from the thirteen Ghost Points.

Disorders of the Anus and External Genitalia

Du 1 is at the junction of the Ren and Du Channels. It is very useful for the anal prolapse, hemorrhoids, prostatitis, genital herpes, vaginitis, and other swelling and pain of the external genitalia.

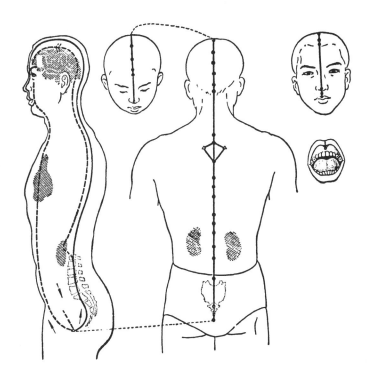

Du Channel

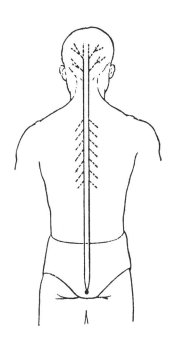

Du Channel Collateral

The Du Channel

督 脉 分 布 圖

The Ren Channel

任 脉

Key Points

- **Ren** means bearing, controlling, and conceiving.
- The Ren Channel regulates all Yin Channels. It is the Sea of Yin Qi.
- The distribution of the Ren Channel is mainly on the central aspect of the abdomen, chest, face, and eye.
- It connects mainly with the uterus, kidney, stomach, spleen, heart, and lung.
- There are 24 points altogether.

The Pathways of the Ren Channel

The Ren Channel has two pathways:

1. Starts below Ren 3, follows the midline of the anterior aspect of the trunk, and passes through the abdomen and chest to the throat, where it meets the Chong Channel. It then goes further up to the face, curves around the lips (intersects Du 28), then up to the area below the eyes (intersects St 1).
2. Starts in the uterus in women, deep inside Ren 4 for men. This is the same starting point as the Du and Chong Channels. It then goes to the perineum (Ren 1) and, together with the Du Channel, goes through the coccyx and penetrates the entire spinal column.

The Associated Organs, Areas, and Points

Ren Channel	
Starting and ending of each pathway	1. Below Ren 3/Below the eyes. 2. Uterus/Spinal Column.
Associated areas of each pathway	1. Lower abdomen, umbilicus, upper abdomen, chest, throat, mouth, lips, and eyes. 2. Uterus, external genitalia, anus, coccyx, and spinal column.
Connected organs	Uterus, kidney, intestines, stomach, spleen, heart, lung, eyes.
Coincides with	Du and Chong Channels
Intersecting points	Du 28, St 1
Confluent and Paired Point	Lu 7, Ki 6

Physiology

The Ren Channel has the following functions:

1. *Regulate all the Yin Channels.* The Ren Channel is called the **Sea of Yin Qi** because all Yin Qi converges in the Ren Channel. There are many aspects of Channel Theory which explain how this occurs: a) The Ren Channel's distribution is mainly on the Yin aspect of the body. b) All six Yin Regular Channels have a connection with the Ren Channel. c) The three Yin Channels of the foot meet with the Ren Channel at Ren 3 and Ren 4. The three Yin Channels of the *Hand* are connected to the Ren channel by virtue of their connection with the three Yin Channels of the *Foot*. d) The Chong Channel intersects the Ren Channel at Ren 7 and Ren 1. The Yin Wei Channel intersects the Ren Channel at the throat (Ren 22, Ren 23), and Yin Qiao Channel meets the Ren Channel through its

connection with the Kidney Channel. This completes the convergence of all Yin Qi in the Ren Channel.

2. *Circulate Yin Qi, including the Blood, Essence, and Body Fluids, to nourish and lubricate all the organs and channels.* Ren Channel points can be used to treat all disorders of the Yin Channels and all syndromes due to either excess or deficiency of Yin Qi. This includes substance deficiency and accumulation. Examples of substances deficiency are those of Blood, Yin, and Essence. Examples of substance accumulation are those of blood stagnation, retention of dampness, stagnation of body fluids, and *Zhen Jia* (masses, tumors, cysts, nodules, and fibroids).

3. *Regulate the reproductive function.* The Ren Channel directly connects with the uterus and external genitalia. The area of Ren 4 and Ren 5, called the *Dantian,* is the location where Essence and *Yuan Qi* (Source Qi) is stored. In women, this is where conception occurs and the fetus is carried. The function of the Ren Channel is more closely associated with women. All the male and female reproductive disorders can be treated by the Ren Channel.

4. *Regulate the function of the internal organs.* Ren Channel's distribution connects with all the internal organs as it passes through the abdomen and chest. It also connects with the internal organs through the Six Yin Channels and the front Mu points, most of which are located on the Ren Channel. In addition, it coincides with the Chong and Du Channels, through which it reaches the Back Shu points. When the Qi of the Ren Channel is obstructed, the Yin Qi will be stagnant, causing disorders of the internal organs, such as pain and spasm, and other dysfunctions.

5. *Distribute the Yin Qi upward to the face, lips, and eyes.* All the Yin Qi accumulates in the Ren Channel, which is then sent directly upward to nourish the sense organs, especially the eyes and lips.

6. *Treat the seven hernias.* Please refer to the chapter on the Liver Channel for a full discussion of the seven hernias.

Pathology

When the Qi of the Ren Channel is disordered there may be irregular menstruation, dysmenorrhea, leukorrhea, seven types of hernia, infertility, vaginal pain, nocturnal emission, enuresis, difficult urination, and pain along the channel distribution.

The Clinical Application of the Ren Channel

The points of the Ren Channel are mainly applied to the disorders of the Zang/Fu organs and reproductive system. It also treats disorders of Yin Qi.

Category	Examples of Symptoms and Signs	Key points in order of importance	Combinations with points from other channels.
Disorders of Yin Qi	• Excess: a) Accumulation of Cold in the interior causing pain and dysfunction	Ren 4, 12, 17	Du 3, UB 23, UB 25, UB 17, Du 12, Sp 4, Pc 6, St 36
	b)Yin substance accumulation: dampness, phlegm, edema, blood stagnation, masses, cysts, fibroids	Ren 12, 9, 5, 4	SJ 4, Lv 3, Sp 6, Sp 9, St 40, UB 22
	• Deficiency: of Blood, Yin, Essence, Body Fluids	Ren 4, 12, 8, 6	UB 17, St 36, Ki 3, Ki 6, GB 39

The Clinical Application of the Ren Channel (continued)

Category	Examples of Symptoms and Signs	Key points in order of importance	Combinations with points from other channels.
Reproductive Disorders	• Female: Infertility, irregular menstruation, dysmenorrhea, leukorrhea, endometriosis, vaginitis, vulvitis, cervicitis.	Ren 4, 3, 2, 1, 5, 24	Sp 6, 4, Pc 6, Lv 3, Lv 5, Lv 8, GB 41, SJ 5, UB 32, UB 23
	• Male: Impotence, nocturnal emission, prostatitis	Ren 4, 6, 3, 1	UB 23, UB 34, Du 3, Sp 6, Ki 3, St 36
Seven Types of Hernia	• Hu Shan - (Fox Hernia), Han Shan - (Cold Hernia), Qi Shan - (Qi Hernia), Tui Shan - (Swelling Hernia), Shui Shan - (Water Hernia), Chong Shan - (Rushing Qi Sensation Hernia), Jing Shan - (Penis Hernia)	Ren 1, 2, 6, 5, 8	Lv 1, St 26, 30, Lv 5, GB 41
Internal organ disorders	• Kidney: Pain in the kidney area, edema, deficiency of essence, Qi, Yin, and Yang.	Ren 4, 5, 9	UB 23, Ki 3, SJ 4, Ren 12, Sp 6
	• Urinary bladder: Painful or difficult urination, retention of urine, enuresis, incontinence.	Ren 3, 4, 6	UB 28, UB 23, GB 25, Sp 9, Lu 7
	• Intestines: Diarrhea, constipation, abdominal distention and pain, flatulence.	Ren 6, 4, 5, 8	St 25, 36, 37, 39, LI 11, Sp 6, UB 25
	• Stomach/spleen: Epigastric pain, nausea, vomiting, indigestion.	Ren 12, 13, 10, 14	St 36, Pc 6, Sp 4, UB 21, 17, Lv 3
	• Lung: Cough, asthma, shortness of breath, stuffiness of the chest	Ren 17, 22, 20	Lu 7, Ki 6, Lu 5, St 40, UB 13
	• Heart: Palpitations, insomnia, dream-disturbed sleep, angina pectoris, anxiety, depression.	Ren 14, 17, 4, 15	Pc 6, Ht 7, Sp 6, UB 15, SI 11
Qi Rushing Up Sensation Syndrome	• Flatulence, asthma, hot flashes and sweating, anxiety attack, palpitations, insomnia, acute stomach pain and distention, or hiatal hernia, constipation, retention of urine.	Ren 4, 24, 17, 10, 13, 15	UB 11, St 37, St 39, Lv 3, Sp 4, Pc 6, Sp 6, Du 1, Du 4
Disorders of the Face and Sense Organs	• Dry throat, swollen and painful throat, stiffness of the tongue, aphasia.	Ren 22, 23	Lu 7, Ki 6, Ht 5, St 40, LI 4, UB 10, Du 15
	• Malar flush, skin discoloration, facial puffiness.	Ren 24, 4, 12, 9	LI 4, LI 11, St 37, Sp 6, Du 4, Ki 6
	• Oral herpes, lip sores.	Ren 12, 24, 10	Sp 6, LI 4, Lv 3, Sp 3
	• Chronic eye disorders.	Ren 4, 6	Lv 3, GB 37, GB 20, Du 4, UB 18

The Luo Collateral of Ren Channel

Luo point: Ren 15
Distribution: After separating from the Ren Channel at Ren 15, it distributes over the entire upper and
                 lower abdomen.
Connection: Upper, lower abdomen, and the Du Channel.

Pathology
Excess: Pain of the skin of the abdomen.
Deficiency: Itching of the skin of the abdomen

Clinical Applications

Emotional and Mental Disorders
Ren 15 has a strong calming effect in cases of severe anxiety, emotional upsets, obsessions, worries, and fears. As one of the Ghost Points, it is also effective for epilepsy and manic-depression. Points used in combination with Ren 15 are Ht 7, Pc 6, Lv 3, Du 20, and GB 15.

Skin Disorders
Ren 15 can be used for skin disorders of the abdomen, such as rashes, pain, itching, due to urticaria, psoriasis, allergy, or toxic effect of drugs and alcohol, as well as internal or external exposure to chemical substances. Points used in combination with Ren 15 are LI 11, LI 4, Sp 10, Sp 6, Lu 7, Ki 9, UB 40, and SI 7.

Channel Disorders
Ren 15 can be used for the disorders of the Du Channel, such as acute lumbar sprain.

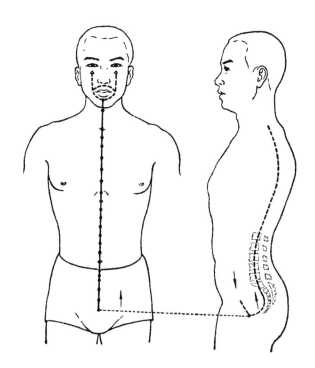

Ren Channel

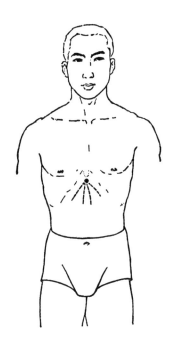

Ren Channel Collateral

The Ren Channel
任 脉 分 布 圖

The Chong Channel
冲 脉

Key Points

- *Chong* has two meanings: 1) the circulation of Blood and Qi with speed and force, like a waterfall, 2) something of strategic importance, as in *Yao Chong*, which means a place of geographically strategic importance.
- The Chong Channel regulates all twelve Regular Channels. It is the Sea of Blood.
- The distribution of the Chong Channel is mainly on the front and back sides of the trunk, face, head, and lower extremities.
- It connects mainly with the uterus, kidney, stomach, heart, and lung.
- Chong Channel has no points of its own. It shares 14 points from other channels. The Sea of Blood points (UB 11, St 37, and St 39) are also considered points of the Chong Channel.

The Pathways of the Chong Channel

The Chong Channel has three pathways:

1. Starts in the lower abdomen, goes to the perineum (intersects Ren 1), emerges at St 30, the *Qi Jie* (*Street of Qi*). It then coincides with the Kidney Channel, ascends through the abdomen (intersects Ki 11, Ki 12, Ki 13, Ki 14), passes around the umbilicus (intersects Ren 7, Ki 15, and Ki 16), then passes through the upper abdomen (intersects Ki 17, Ki 18, Ki 19, Ki 20, Ki 21), and disperses in the chest. From there, it ascends to the throat (Ren 23 area) where the left and right channels converge. It then continues upward to the face, curves around the lips, enters the nasopharynx, and permeates the entire face.
2. Starts from the lower abdomen and connects with the kidney, emerges at St 30 (Qi Jie), descends along the medial aspect of the thigh to the popliteal fossa. From there, it parallels the Kidney Channel traversing the margin of the tibia and the posterior aspect of the medial malleolus, and enters the heel before ending on the sole of the foot. A branch separates above the medial malleolus, crosses the dorsum of the foot following the space between the first and second metatarsals to Tai Chong[1] (Lv 3), and finally reaches the lateral aspect of the big toe.
3. Starts from the uterus in women and deep inside Ren 4 for men, which is the same starting point as for the Du and Ren Channels. From there, it inclines backward to enter the spine, and circulates through the spinal column following the Du Channel.

The Associated Organs, Areas, and Points

Chong Channel	
Starting and ending of each pathway	1. Lower abdomen; emerges around St 30 (Qi Jie)/Face 2. Lower abdomen; emerges around St 30 (Qi Jie)/Sole of the foot and big toe 3. Uterus/Spinal column

---

[1] Tai Chong is another name used for the Chong Channel and also the name of the point Lv 3. The pulse on this point is used to diagnose the excess or deficiency of Chong Channel.

The Associated Organs, Areas, and Points (continued)

Chong Channel	
Associated areas of each pathway	1. Lower abdomen, Qi Jie, upper abdomen, chest, throat, lips, nasopharynx, face. 2. Kidney, Qi Jie, medial aspect of the lower extremities, posterior aspect of the medial malleolus, heel, sole of the foot, dorsum of the foot, big toe. 3. Uterus, spinal column.
Connected organs	Kidney, uterus, heart, stomach, lung, throat, nasopharynx
Coincides with	Kidney and Du Channel
Points (intersecting points)	St 30, Ki 11, Ki 12, Ki 13, Ki 14, Ren 7, Ki 15, Ki 16, Ki 17, Ki 18, Ki 19, Ki 20, Ki 21, Ren 1 KD 11-21
Confluent and Paired Point	Sp 4, Pc 6
Sea of Blood Points	UB 11, St 37, 39

Physiology

The Chong Channel has the following functions:

1. *Store and regulate the blood.* The Chong Channel is the **Sea of Blood**. Blood is produced in the middle Jiao and from Kidney Essence. They are considered the source of Blood. The Chong Channel coincides with the Kidney Channel and intersects the Stomach Channel at St 30. The Chong Channel is directly related to the functions of the Blood.

   a) The Chong Channel is effective for treating all disorders related to the blood including deficiency, excess, heat, and cold. In women, Blood is considered the primary material basis for their physiological functions. The Chong Channel is directly connected with the uterus which is called the **Mansion of Blood**. Clinically, the Chong Channel is effective for gynecological and obstetrical disorders such as dysmenorrhea, irregular menstruation, infertility, miscarriage, and difficult delivery.

   b) The Chong Channel curves around the lips. It is also related to the pubic region and perineum. The distribution of hair in those areas results from abundant circulation of Blood in the Chong Channel. Women do not develop significant amounts of facial hair because their frequent blood loss through menstruation creates a relative state of Blood Deficiency. If a woman develops facial hair or a sparse distribution of pubic hair, it indicates a disorder of the Blood and of the Chong Channel. In western medical terms, this is a hormone imbalance.

2. *Regulate the Twelve Regular Channels.* The Chong Channel is the Sea of the Twelve Channels. It coincides with the Du Channel and intersects the Ren Channel. It shares their functions of controlling and regulating all Twelve Regular Channels. The Chong Channel is the most powerfully effective channel for regulating the circulation Qi and Blood in the entire body. It treats **Rebellion of Qi**, which usually manifest along the pathways of the Chong Channel. Symptoms manifested include a the sensation of Qi rushing upward in the chest, throat, and head, as well as hot flashes and cramping pain of the abdomen.

   The Chong Channel by virtue of its function of promoting circulation of Qi and Blood, is the most powerful channel for opening blockages and stagnations, including such extreme cases as gangrene, severe neuropathies, Raynaud's disease, masses, and edema. Both the Ren and Chong Channels are effective for the treatment of accumulations and masses. However, the Ren Channel is more effectively applied in those instances where the original cause was Qi stagnation, while Chong Channel is more effective for those due to Blood disorders.

Pathology

When the Chong Channel is disordered, there may be Blood disorders of either excess or deficiency. In Blood excess conditions, heat and stagnation may develop in the blood. There may be a sense of fullness and distention of the body, as if it were enlarge. The Blood circulation is accelerated and stagnated. There may also be agitation and a flushed face due to Qi and Blood rushing to the head. Hypertension and menopause are two possible examples of this type of disorder. In Blood deficiency conditions, there may be general weakness, coldness of the body, a sensation as if the body were being reduced in size, and retarded circulation. Symptoms and signs of the Chong Channel also include irregular menstruation, dysmenorrhea, miscarriage, infertility, difficulty delivery, impotence, sensations of Qi rushing upward to the chest, throat, and head, cramping pain of the abdomen, severe, acute onset of all types of bleeding, asthma, dizziness, headache, and vomiting.

The Clinical Applications of the Chong Channel

The points of the Chong Channel are mainly applied to the disorders of the reproductive system. It also treats disorders of Qi and Blood. According to Channel Theory, the Stomach Channel dominates the disorders of Blood, and the San Jiao Channel dominates the disorders of Qi. The Chong Channel is also used to treat disorders of both Qi and Blood, but primarily those symptoms caused by rebellion of Qi and Blood.

Category	Examples of Symptoms and Signs	Key points in order of importance	Combinations with points from other channels.
Disorders of the Reproductive System	• Menstruation: irregular menstruation, dysmenorrhea, endometriosis, amenorrhea, menorrhagia, metrorrhagia, menopause, PMS	Sp 4, UB 11, St 37, St 39, Ren 7, Ki 11-16	Pc 6, Ren 4, Lv 3, LI 4, Sp 6, Sp 10, Sp 1, UB 23, SJ 4, Shiqizhuixia, UB 32
	• Pregnancy: infertility, miscarriage, morning sickness, abdominal pain with bleeding, toxemia of pregnancy.	Sp 4, UB 11, St 37, 39, Ren 7, Ki 11-16	Pc 6, Zigong, Lv 3, UB 23, Ren 12, SJ 4, St 36
	• Delivery and post-partum: difficult labor, retained placenta, post-partum bleeding, depression	Sp 4, UB 11, St 37, 39,	LI 4, Sp 6, UB 67, UB 60
	• Abnormal vaginal discharge: abnormal color or quantity, leukorrhea with itching or pain.	Sp 4, UB 11, St 37, 39, Ren 7, Ki 11	Lv 5, Ren 3, Lv 3, Sp 9, SJ 5, GB 41, GB 26
	• Breast: insufficient lactation, mastitis, fibrocystic mastitis	Sp 4, St 37, 39, Ki 23	SI 1, Ren 17, SI 11, St 40, Pc 6
	• Pelvic inflammatory disease, adnexitis, genital herpes, inflammation of the external genitalia	St 30, Ren 1, Ki 11-16	Lv 5, Lv 3, St 28, UB 32, SJ 5, GB 41
	• Men: Impotence, nocturnal emission sterility, spermatorrhea, inflammation of the external genitalia, genital herpes, hernia.	Sp 4, Ren 7, Ren 1, Ki 11-16, St 30	Ren 4, Sp 6, Ki 3, 6, Lv 3, SJ 4, 5, Lv 1, Lv 3, Lv 5, GB 41

The Clinical Applications of the Chong Channel (continued)

Category	Examples of Symptoms and Signs	Key points in order of importance	Combinations with points from other channels.
Disorders of Qi and Blood	• <u>Blood Deficiency:</u> Anemia, dizziness, palpitations, insomnia, pale complexion, cold sensation, body feels like it is shrinking.	Sp 4, UB 11, St 37, St 39, Ki 16	St 36, Ren 6, UB 15, UB 17, UB 19, UB 20, UB 23
	• <u>Blood Excess</u> Blood stagnation, hot sensation of the body, body feels expanded, over-excitement, over-stimulation.	St 30, UB 11, St 37, St 39	LI 11, SJ 5, Du 14, Sp 6
	• <u>Rebellion of Qi and Blood:</u> *Acute bleeding*: epistaxis, hemoptysis, hematemesis, menorrhagia, metrorrhagia, hematuria, purpura hematochezia,	St 30, UB 11, St 37, St 39, Sp 4	Lu 6, Pc 4, Sp 1, GB 34, Ki 5, Ki 3, Lv 3
	Blood blockage: gangrene, severe neuropathies, arteriosclerosis, atherosclerosis, thrombosis	St 30, UB 11, St 37, St 39, Sp 4, Ki 13, Ki 16	St 42, Lv 3, GB 34, St 40, Sp 9, Sp 6, LI 11
	Qi rushing up to the chest: acute asthma, suffocating sensation in the chest, dyspnea, palpitations, restlessness, anxiety.	St 30, UB 11, St 37, St 39, Sp 4, Ki 13	Pc 6, Ren 17, Lu 6, Pc 4, Ki 4
	Qi rushing up to the throat: sudden hoarseness, sudden aphasia, acute Plum-Pit Qi Syndrome	St 30, UB 11, St 37, St 39, Sp 4, Ki 13	Pc 6, Ht 5, Ren 22, Ren 17, St 40
	Qi rushing up to the head: dizziness, vertigo, light-headedness, throbbing headache, blurring of vision, flushed face	St 30, UB 11, St 37, St 39, Sp 4, Ki 13	Lv 3, 2, LI 4, Pc 6, SJ 5, Sp 6
	Qi rushing up to the Stomach: epigastric distention, abdominal cramps, vomiting, nausea, hiccup, frequent belching.	Sp 4, St 30, UB 11, St 37, St 39, Ki 13, Ki 16, Ki 19	Pc 6, Ren 10, St 36, UB 17, St 25, Sp 6
Disorders of the Endocrine system	• Hyperthyroidism, hypothyroidism, adrenal cortical insufficiency, pituitary insufficiency, diabetes	UB 11, St 37, St 39, Sp 4, Ren 7, Ki 13, Ki 16, St 30	Ren 12, SJ 4, LI 4, SJ 10, Ki 3, Du 4, Sp 6, St 36
Zhen Jia (masses)	• Masses, tumors, nodules, cysts, fibroids, edema, dampness and phlegm accumulations	Sp 4, UB 11, St 37, 39, Ki 13, 14, St 30	Ren 12, SJ 4, 5, St 40, Sp 9, LI 4, Lv 3, GB 30, UB 22
Wei syndrome	• Paralysis, flaccidity and weakness of the muscles especially the lower extremities	UB 11, St 37, St 39, St 30	GB 26, St 36, 32, GB 34, LI 15, LI 11, LI 4, Lv 3

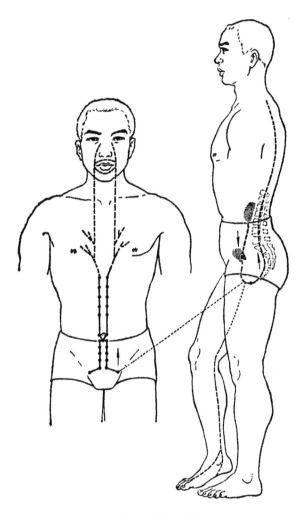

Chong Channel

The Chong Channel
冲 脉 分 布 圖

The Dai Channel

Key Points

- *Dai* means girdle or belt.
- The Dai Channel is the only channel which circulates transversely, like a belt to bind and control all the channels which run longitudinally.
- The distribution of Dai Channel circles the waist.
- It connects mainly with the kidney and uterus.
- Dai Channel has no points of its own. It shares 3 points from the Gall Bladder Channel.

The Pathway of the Dai Channel

The Dai Channel starts between the second and third lumbar vertebrae(intersects Du 4), where it is directly connected with the Kidney Divergent Channel. It circulates continuously without ending, covering the area of the waist and umbilicus (intersects GB 26, GB 27, and GB 28). The ancient text, Qi Jing Ba Mai Kao (Research on the Eight Extraordinary Channels) states that Lv 13 is the starting point of the Dai Channel.

The Associated Organs, Areas, and Points

Dai Channel	
Starts/Ends	From Du 4 (Kidney Divergent Channel); it circulates endlessly.
Associated areas	Lumbar vertebrae, waist, hypochondriac region, umbilicus.
Connected organs	Kidney, uterus
Coincides with	None
Points (intersecting points)	GB 26, GB 27, GB 28
Confluent and Paired Point	GB 41, SJ 5
Related points	Du 4, Lv 13, Ren 8

Physiology

The Dai Channel has the following functions:
1. *Control and bind all the channels which travel longitudinally.* Dai Channel is the only channel which circulates transversely. It binds and controls the Du, Ren, Chong, Yin/Yang Wei and Yin/Yang Qiao Channels and all six Regular Channels of the Foot, and through them, connects with the six Regular Channels of the Hand. The Dai channel is directly derived from the Kidney Divergent Channel and circulates around the waist. Its function is to regulate the areas of the waist, lumbar spine, and lower extremities. Symptoms such as lower back pain with coldness, weakness, and flaccidity, as well as paralysis of the lower extremities, are considered disorders of the Dai Channel.
2. *Regulate leukorrhea.* The word Dai also has the meaning of "leukorrhea," indicating the channel's direct connection with the uterus. The Dai Channel is effective for treating abnormal vaginal discharge, disorders of the external genitalia, and menstruation.
3. *Regulate the Gall Bladder Channel.* The Dai Channel is directly related to the Gall Bladder Channel through its Confluent Point (GB 41) and to the waist (GB 26, GB 27, and GB 28 are its other shared points). It is effective for regulating the Gall Bladder Channel, especially disorders which appear on

the sides of the body. Disorders such as migraine headache, ear, neck, and Shao Yang Syndrome can be treated by Dai Channel points.

Pathology

When the Dai Channel is disordered, there may be muscle weakness and flaccidity or paralysis of the lower extremities, abdominal distention and fullness, abdominal obesity, lower back pain, and leukorrhea.

The Clinical Applications of the Dai Channel

The points of Dai Channel are mainly used for abnormal vaginal discharge, and the disorders of the lower back, lumbar region, abdomen, waist, and lower extremities. It can also be used to treat the disorders of the Gall Bladder Channel.

Category	Examples of Symptoms and Signs	Key points in order of importance	Combinations with points from other channels.
Bi and Wei Syndromes	• Lower back pain with coldness • Weakness, flaccidity or paralysis of the extremities • Spasm, numbness, and pain of the four extremities	GB 26, 41 GB 26, 27, 28, 41 GB 26, 41	Du 4, UB 23, Ki 3 St 36, St 32, GB 34, LI 11 Lv 3, GB 34, SJ 5, Sp 3
Disorders of the Abdomen	• Abdominal fullness and distention, which may refer to the lower back, flatulence, borborygmus, ascites, abdominal obesity, masses	GB 26, 28, 41	Lv 13, St 36, 37, Sp 6, Sp 9, Ki 4

Disorders of Urogenital system	• Abnormal vaginal discharge
	  Excess: Yellow or white with increased quantity, odor.
	  Deficiency: Dilute, continuous discharge.
	• Metrorrhagia, menorrhagia, irregular menstruation, prolapse of the uterus
	• Retention of urine, enuresis, incontinence.
	• Eczema, herpes of the external genitalia.
		GB 41, 26, 27, 28
		
		GB 26, 41
		
		GB 26, 41, 28
		
		GB 41, 26
		
		GB 41, 26
			Lv 2, Lv 3, Lv 5, Lv 8, Sp 9, Sp 6, SJ 5, SJ 6, UB 32
			Du 4, UB 23, Ren 4
			
			Sp 1, GB 34, St 36, Lv 3, Lv 8, Sp 6, Ren 4
			Ren 3, Sp 6, Sp 9, Lu 7, Ki 6, UB 23
			SJ 5, Lv 5, Lv 2, Ren 1, Ren 2, Ren 3, St 36, LI 11

Disorders of Gall Bladder Channel	• Migraine headache, redness and pain of the eyes, mumps, lymph gland swellings, deafness, tinnitus, hypochondriac pain, pulling sensation of one side of the body, Shao Yang Syndrome.	GB 41, 26	SJ 5, SJ 3, Lv 3, GB 34, GB 20, Sp 6

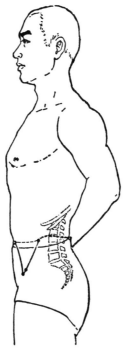

Dai Channel

The Dai Channel

帶 脉 分 布 圖

The Yin Qiao and Yang Qiao Channels
陰蹺脉、陽蹺脉

Key Points
* *Qiao* means the heel and the movement of the foot.
* The Yin/Yang Qiao Channels balance the Yin/Yang Qi of the body. This includes the balance of the medial and lateral aspects of the lower extremities, and the opening and closing of the eyes.
* The distribution of Yang Qiao Channel is mainly on the lateral side of the lower extremities, hip, hypochondriac region, shoulder, face, inner canthus, and to the brain. The distribution of the Yin Qiao Channel is mainly on the medial aspect of the lower extremities, external genitalia, abdomen, chest, throat, face, inner canthus, and to the brain.
* The Yang Qiao Channel connects with the brain. The Yin Qiao Channel connects with the external genitalia and the brain.
* Neither Yin Qiao nor Yang Qiao Channels have any points of their own. Yang Qiao Channel shares 13 points with other channels. Yin Qiao Channel shares 3 points with other channels.

The Pathway of the Yang Qiao Channel

The Yang Qiao Channel begins below the external malleolus (intersects UB 62 and UB 61), ascends the lateral aspect of the leg (intersects UB 59) and thigh to the hip (intersects GB 29), then passes through the lateral aspect of the abdomen and hypochondiac region. From there, it travels to the lateral aspect of the scapula and shoulder (intersects SI 10, LI 16, and LI 15), follows the lateral side of the neck to the corner of the mouth (intersects St 4, St 3, and St 1), then goes to the inner canthus (intersects UB 1) where it joins the Yin Qiao, Urinary Bladder, and many other channels[1]. From there, the Yin/Yang Qiao Channels ascend the forehead, go laterally along the side of the head (intersects GB 20), and finally enter the brain (intersects Du 16).

The Pathway of the Yin Qiao Channel

The Yin Qiao Channel starts below the medial malleolus (intersects Ki 6) and extends upward along the medial aspect of the leg (intersects Ki 8) and thigh, passes through the external genitalia, where it enters the body cavity. It then travels internally through the abdomen, up to the chest before emerging at the supraclavicular fossa. From there, it ascends through the throat, passes through St 9, goes to the face, then through the zygomatic arch, and joins the Yang Qiao Channel at the inner canthus (intersects UB 1). From there, the Yin/Yang Qiao Channels ascend the forehead, go laterally along the side of the head, and finally enter the brain.

---

[1] See Section IV. The Channel System's Relationship with the Organs and Other Body Structures, in the Theory of Channel and Collaterals section.

The Associated Organs, Areas and Points

Yin/Yang Qiao		
Starts/Ends	Yang Qiao:	UB 62/Du 16, brain
	Yin Qiao:	Ki 6/Du 16, brain
Associated areas	Yang Qiao:	External malleolus, lateral aspect of the lower extremities, hip, hypochondriac region, lateral aspect of scapula and shoulder, face, inner canthus, side of the head, and the brain.
	Yin Qiao:	Medial malleolus, medial aspect of the lower extremities, external genitalia, abdomen, chest, throat, face, inner canthus, side of the head, and the brain.
Connected organs	Yang Qiao:	Eye, brain
	Yin Qiao:	Eye, brain
Coincides with	None	
Points (intersecting points)	Yang Qiao:	UB 62, UB 61, UB 59, GB 29, SI 10, LI 16, LI 15 St 4, St 3, St 1, UB 1, GB 20, Du 16
	Yin Qiao:	Ki 6, Ki 8, UB 1
Confluent and Paired Points	Yang Qiao:	UB 62, SI 3
	Yin Qiao:	Ki 6, Lu 7

Physiology

The functions of the Yin and Yang Qiao Channels can be summarized as follows:

1. *Balance the Yin/Yang Qi of the lower extremities.* This includes the muscular balance of the medial and lateral aspects of the leg, and actions of inversion and eversion of the foot. If the medial muscles are spasmed, causing a pulling sensation, and the lateral muscles are flaccid or paralyzed, this is a disorder of the Yin Qiao. If the lateral muscles are spasmed, and the medial muscles are flaccid or paralyzed, this is a disorder of Yang Qiao.

2. *Regulate the opening and closing of the eyes.* Both the Yin and Yang Qiao Channels go to the inner canthus and control the normal circulatory cycle of the Yin Qi and Yang Qi. If the Yang Qi is in excess, the eyes remain open resulting in insomnia. If the Yin Qi is in excess, the result is somnolence. Eye disorders such as redness and pain of the inner canthus, iritis, optic nerve atrophy, and glaucoma, can also be treated with points of the Yin/Yang Qiao Channels.

3. *Regulate the function of the brain.* Both the Yin/Yang Qiao Channels go to the brain and greatly influence its function. When Yang Qi is in excess in the Yang Qiao Channel, there will be over-excitement, hyperactivity, restlessness, and uneasiness. When Yin Qi is in excess in the Yin Qiao Channel, there will be spiritlessness, hypoactivity, apathy, and lassitude. Clinically, Yin/Yang Qiao Channels can be used to treat mental, emotional, and brain disorders, such as epilepsy, convulsions, tremors, manic-depression, and schizophrenia.

4. It is said that the Yang Qiao Channel is a branch of the Urinary Bladder Channel. Therefore, symptoms of the Urinary Bladder Channel can be treated by Yang Qiao points. Some examples include pain and stiffness of the back, neck, shoulder, spinal column, joints and bones, as well as aversion to wind, headache, sweating, epistaxis, and numbness and coldness of the hands and feet. It is said that the Yin Qiao Channel is a branch of the Kidney Channel. Therefore, the symptoms of the Kidney Channel can be treated by the Yin Qiao Channel. These include pain of the lower and lateral abdomen, hip joint or lumbar pain referring to the external genitalia, hernia, uterine bleeding, dribbling or painful urination, borborygmus, diarrhea and constipation, and abdominal masses. The

Yin Qiao Channel also passes through the throat. It is therefore used for disorders of the throat and vocal cords.

Pathology

Yang Qiao Channel

When the Yang Qiao Channel is disordered, there may be insomnia, epilepsy, muscle spasms on the lateral aspect of the lower extremities while those on the medial aspect may be flaccid or atrophied. There may also be eversion of the foot, and pain and stiffness of the lumbar region, hip, scapula, shoulder, and headache.

Yin Qiao Channel

When the Yin Qiao Channel is disordered, there may be somnolence, epilepsy, muscle spasm on the medial aspect of the lower extremities while those on the lateral aspect may be flaccid or atrophied. There may also be inversion of the foot, lower abdominal and lumbar pain, pain in the external genitalia, hernia, leukorrhea, and sore throat.

The Clinical Applications of the Yin Qiao and Yang Qiao Channels

The points of both the Yin/Yang Qiao Channels are mainly used for the disorders affecting the movement of the muscles of the lower extremities. They can also be used to treat sleeping disorders and epilepsy. The points of Yang Qiao Channel are used for hyperactive mental disorders, such as Kuang syndrome, over-excitement, and restlessness. The points of the Yin Qiao Channel are used for hypoactive mental disorders, such as depression, spiritlessness, apathy, and lassitude

Category	Examples of Symptoms and Signs	Key points in order of importance	Combinations points from other channels.
Channel Obstruction	• Yang Qiao: Lateral muscle spasms, loosening of the medial muscles, eversion of the foot.	UB 62, Ki 6, UB 59	SI 3, Lv 3, GB 34, St 36
	Pain, stiffness, and difficult movement of the back, shoulder, scapula and neck, headache, general pain of the joints and bones, aversion to wind, sweating, epistaxis, numbness and coldness of the hands and feet.	UB 62, UB 59, GB 29, SI 10, LI 15	SI 3, LI 10, UB 40, GB 34, Lv 3, UB 23, Du 3, Du 9
	• Yin Qiao: Medial muscle spasms, loosening of the lateral muscles, inversion of the foot.	Ki 6, UB 62, Ki 8	Lu 7, Lv 3, GB 34, Sp 6, Lv 8
Sleeping disorders	• Yang Qiao excess or Yin Qiao deficiency: Insomnia	UB 62, Ki 6, GB 20	Ht 7, Pc 6, Sp 6, UB 15
	• Yin Qiao excess or Yang Qiao deficiency: Somnolence	Ki 6, UB 62	Du 20, Sp 3, St 40
Eye disorders	• Pain and redness of the inner canthus, iritis, optic nerve atrophy, glaucoma.	Ki 6, UB 62, UB 1, GB 20	Lv 3, GB 37, LI 11, SI 6

The Clinical Applications of the Yin Qiao and Yang Qiao Channels (continued)

Category	Examples of Symptoms and Signs	Key points in order of importance	Combinations points from other channels.
Disorders of the brain, mind, and emotions	• Yin/Yang Qiao: epilepsy, convulsions, tremors, manic-depression, schizophrenia.	UB 62, Ki 6, GB 20, Du 16	Lv 2, 3 LI 4, St 40, selection of 13 Ghost Points
	• Yang Qiao: over-excitement, hyperactivity, restlessness and uneasiness.	UB 62, Ki 6, GB 20, Du 16	LI 4, Lv 3, Pc 6, Sp 6
	• Yin Qiao: spiritlessness, hypoactivity, apathy and lassitude.	Ki 6, UB 62, GB 20	Du 20, SJ 3, Ki 4, UB 52, UB 44
Disorders of the lower abdomen (intestinal/uro-genital)	• Yin Qiao: Lower, lateral abdominal pain, hernia, pain of the external genitalia, referring to the hip and lumbar region and vice versa, uterine bleeding, irregular menstruation, unsmooth and dribbling urination, borborygmus, diarrhea and constipation, abdominal masses.	Ki 6, Ki 8, GB 29	Lv 2, Lv 3, Ren 2, Ren 3, 4, GB 26, UB 23, Du 4, St 30
Disorders of the throat and vocal cords	• Yin Qiao: Chronic pharyngitis, laryngitis, weak voice, nodules on the vocal cords, hoarse voice, Plum Pit Qi syndrome	Ki 6	Lu 7, Ht 5, Lu 10, St 40, Ren 23, St 9, Pc 6,

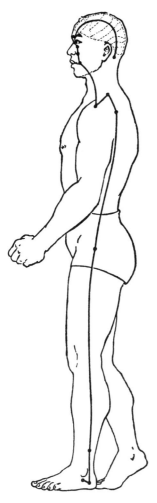

Yangqiao Channel

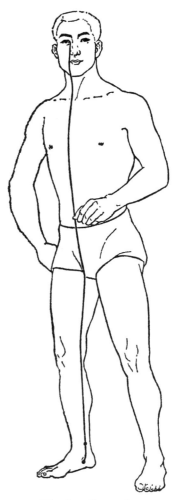

Yinqiao Channel

The Yangqiao and Yinqiao Channels
陽 蹻 脈 、 陰 蹻 脈 分 布 圖

The Yin Wei and Yang Wei Channels
陰 維 脉、陽 維 脉

Key Points

- *Wei* means connecting; making a network; gathering the other channels together.
- The Yin and Yang Wei Channels connect all the Yin and Yang Channels respectively.
- The distribution of the Yang Wei Channel is mainly on the lateral aspect of the lower extremities, the hypochondriac region, the lateral side of the shoulder, retroauricular area, forehead, lateral side of the head, and the nape (where it meets with the Du Channel).

  The distribution of the Yin Wei Channel is mainly on the medial aspect of the lower extremities, abdomen, hypochondriac region, diaphragm, chest, throat, and root of the tongue (where it meets with the Ren Channel).
- Yang Wei Channel connects with the ear and brain. The Yin Wei Channel connects with the throat and tongue
- The Yin Wei and Yang Wei Channels have no points of their own. Yang Wei Channel shares 16 points with other channels. The Yin Wei Channel shares 8 points with other channels.

The Pathway of the Yang Wei Channel

The Yang Wei Channel starts at the lateral aspect of the foot (intersects UB 63). It follows the pathway of the Gall Bladder Channel upward on the lateral aspect of the lower extremities (intersects GB 35) to the hip joint. It then travels further upward to the hypochondriac region, through the posterior aspect of the shoulder (intersects SI 10 and SJ 15), up the neck (intersects GB 21) to the retroauricular area and the forehead (intersects St 8). From there, it reaches to the back of the head (intersects GB 13 - GB 20) and ends at the nape, where it intersects with the Du Channel (intersects Du 15 and Du 16). It should also be noted that the Nan Jing (Classic of Difficulties) says that the Yang Wei Channel starts from the meeting point of the Yang Channels of foot, GB 35 (Yang Jiao).

The Pathway of the Yin Wei Channel

The Yin Wei Channel originates from the medial aspect of the lower leg (intersects Ki 9). It follows the medial aspect of the leg, knee, and thigh, then goes to the lateral abdomen (intersects Sp 12, Sp 13, Sp 15, and Sp 16) and the hypochondriac region (intersects Lv 14). It passes through the diaphragm and chest, then goes to the sides of the throat (intersects Ren 22 and Ren 23) and the root of the tongue. The Nan Jing (Classic of Difficulties) says that the Yin Wei Channel starts from the meeting point of the Yin Channels of foot, Sp 6, whose name *Sanyinjiao* means "three Yin meeting".

The Associated Organs, Areas and Points

Yin/Yang Wei		(intersects) (starts)
Starts/Ends	Yang Wei: Yin Wei:	UB 63; (GB 35)/nape (Du 16) Ki 9; (Sp 6) /root of tongue (Ren 23)
Associated areas	Yang Wei: Yin Wei: aspect throat,	Lateral side of the lower extremities, hip, hypochondriac region, lateral side of the shoulder, neck, retroauricular area, forehead, side of the head, nape. Medial aspect of the lower extremities, lateral of the abdomen, hypochondriac region, chest, tongue.
Connected organs	Yang Wei: Yin Wei:	Ear, brain Throat, tongue
Coincides with	Yang Wei: Yin Wei:	Gall Bladder Channel Spleen Channel
Points (intersecting points)	Yang Wei: GB 13-20 Yin Wei:	UB 63, GB 35, SI 10, SJ 15, GB 21, St 8, GB 13, GB 14, GB 15, GB 16, GB 17, GB 18, GB 19, GB 20, Du 15, Du 16 Ki 9, (Sp 6)[1], Sp 12, Sp 13, Sp 15, Sp 16, Lv 14, Ren 22, Ren 23
Confluent and Paired Points	Yang Wei: Yin Wei:	SJ 5, GB 41 P 6, Sp 4

Physiology

The Yin/Yang Wei Channels connect and regulate all Yin/Yang Channels of the body. Yang Wei Channel dominates the exterior, while the Yin Wei Channel dominates the interior. They should balance each other. Their functions are summarized as follows:

Yang Wei Channel:
1. *Dominate the exterior.* Yang Wei Channel regulates the Qi in the Yang Channels, especially the Tai Yang and Shao Yang Channels. Symptoms of the Tai Yang Channels, such as aversion to cold, fever, headache, obstruction of the nose, and floating pulse, can be considered disorders of Yang Wei Channel. Symptoms of Shao Yang Syndrome, such as alternating chills and fever, distention and fullness of the hypochondriac region and chest, bitter taste in the mouth, poor appetite, and wiry pulse, can be treated by Yang Wei channel.
2. *Balance the Yang Qi.* When Yang Qi is in excess, there may be symptoms such as dizziness, vertigo, blurred vision, asthmatic breathing. When Yang Qi is deficient, there may be symptoms such as general lassitude, and listlessness. Yang Wei Channel points are appropriate for treating both excess and deficiency of Yang Qi.
3. *Balance the emotions.* When the Qi in the Yang Channels is disturbed, there may be manic-depression, obsessive/compulsive behavior, and excessive anger. In these cases, Yang Wei Channel points can be applied to reestablish the balance.

---

[1] See above note and reference to the Nan Jing (Classic of Difficulties)

Yin Wei Channel:

1. *Dominates the interior.* The Yin Wei Channel dominates the Qi in the Yin Channels and their associated organs, especially the heart, lung, stomach, and spleen. Disorders and symptoms of those organs such as chest pain, cardiac and epigastric pain, pain of the abdomen and external genitalia, fullness and distention in the hypochondriac region, abdominal masses, borborygmus, diarrhea, or lumbar pain can be treated with Yin Wei Channel points.
2. *Balance the emotions.* When the Qi in the Yin Channels is disturbed, there may be mental instability, uneasiness, low self esteem, lack of will power, and discouragement. In these cases, Yin Wei points can be applied to lift the spirit and balance the emotions.

The Comparison of the Regulatory Functions of Ren/Du Channel, the Yin/Yang Qiao and Yin/Yang Wei Channels.

It has been said that the Ren/Du, Yin/Yang Qiao and Yin/Yang Wei Channels have regulatory functions for all Yin and Yang Channels. The Ren/Du Channels have general balancing functions, while those of the Yin/Yang Qiao and Yin/Yang Wei Channels are more specific. The Yin/Yang Qiao Channels mainly balance the medial and lateral aspects of the lower extremities, and include many functions of the Urinary Bladder and Kidney Channels. The Yin/Yang Wei Channels mainly balance the interior and exterior and include many functions of the Gall Bladder and Spleen Channels.

Pathology

When the Yang Wei Channel is disordered there may be exterior syndromes, vertigo, chills, and fever alternately, muscular stiffness and pain, fatigue, pain, and distention in the waist. When the Yin Wei Channel is disordered, there may be interior syndromes, cardiac pain, pain of the stomach, chest, or abdomen.

The Clinical Applications of the Yin Wei and Yang Wei Channels

The points of the Yang Wei Channel are mainly used to treat exterior syndromes, Shao Yang syndrome, and symptoms related to the Gall Bladder Channel. The points of the Yin Wei Channel are mainly used to treat interior syndromes and disorders of the heart, chest, and stomach.

The Clinical Applications of the Yin Wei and Yang Wei Channels (continued)

Category	Examples of Symptoms and Signs	Key points in order of importance	Combinations with points from other channels.
Yang Wei Disorders	• Tai Yang Syndromes: Wind Cold and Wind Heat.	SJ 5, UB 63, Du 16, GB 20	UB 62, SI 3, UB 12, Lu 7
	• Shao Yang Syndromes: chills and fever alternately, chest and hypochondriac discomfort, bitter taste in the mouth.	SJ 5, GB 20, 14, GB 35	GB 41, LI 4, LI 11, Lv 3
	• Yang Qi excess: febrile diseases, hyperactivity of Yang Qi.	SJ 5, GB 20, GB 30, UB 63	GB 41, Lv 2, Lv 3, LI 11
	• Yang Qi deficiency: general lassitude, cold.	SJ 5	Du 4, Du 14, Du 20, St 36
	• Emotional disorders: manic-depression, obsessive/compulsive behavior, and excessive anger.	SJ 5, GB 13, GB 15, GB 20, Du 16	Lv 2, GB 41, St 40, selection from 13 Ghost Points
	• Channel obstruction (mainly Gall Bladder Channel): pain of the joints and bones, eyes, pain of the hip, hypochondriac region, and neck.	SJ 5, GB 35, 14, SJ 15, GB 21	GB 41, 39, Lv 3, UB 11, UB 65
Yin Wei Disorders	• Heart, chest and stomach disorders: cardiac pain, chest stuffiness, epigastric pain, vomiting, borborygmus, diarrhea, abdominal masses.	Pc 6, Lv 14, Sp 9	Sp 4, Ren 12, Ren 17, LI 4, Lv 3, St 36
	• Emotional disorders: mental instability, uneasiness, low self esteem, lack of will power and discouragement.	Pc 6, Sp 9, Lv 14	Lv 3, Ht 7, GB 41, UB 52, 15, Du 20
Disharmony of Yin/Yang Wei Channels	• Epilepsy, mutism	Du 15, Du 16, SJ 5, GB 20	Du 2, Ren 15, UB 62, Ki 6

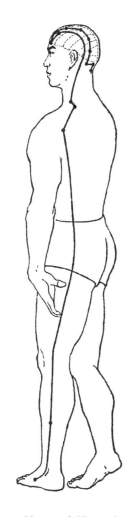

Yangwei Channel

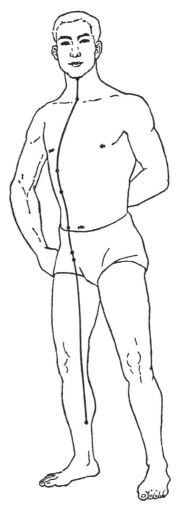

Yinwei Channel

The Yangwei and Yinwei Channels

陽 維 脉 、 陰 維 脉 分 布 圖

Summary and Comparison of the Eight Extraordinary Channels

Among the Eight Extraordinary Channels, there are three Sea Channels. The Du Channel is the Sea of Yang Qi, and mainly distributes on the back of the body. The Ren Channel is the Sea of Yin Qi, and mainly distributes on the front of the body. The Chong Channel is the Sea of Blood and Twelve Channels, and its distribution covers the whole body. The Dai Channel regulates all channels which run longitudinally. The Du, Ren, Chong, and Dai Channels all derive their energy from the Kidney. The Yin/Yang Qiao Channels control and balance the left and right sides of the body, while the Yin/Yang Wei Channels balance the interior and exterior aspects. Together, the Eight Extraordinary Channels make a network which integrates the Twelve Channel System. They serve as a reservoir to store and distribute Qi and Blood to the whole body.

Channel	Main areas of distribution	Connected Channels/Organs	Functions	Pathology
Du	Perineum, external genitalia, anus, midline of the back and head, spinal column, nose, inner canthus, upper lip	• Ren, Urinary Bladder, Chong and Kidney Channels • Kidney, brain, uterus	Sea of Yang Qi Govern all Yang Channels.	Disorders of Yang Qi, rigidity and stiffness of the spinal column, opisthotonos, epilepsy, convulsions, hemorrhoids.
Ren	Perineum, external genitalia, anus, midline of the abdomen and chest, throat, lips, eyes	• Du, Chong, Kidney and Stomach Channels • Uterus, kidney	Sea of Yin Qi Controlling all Yin Channels Dominate the function of the uterus and pregnancy.	Disorders of Yin Qi, irregular menstruation, infertility, leukorrhea, hernia, difficult urination, enuresis, nocturnal emission, vaginal pain.
Chong	Perineum, abdomen, chest, throat, lips, eye Medial aspect of the lower extremities, dorsum of the foot Spinal column	• Kidney, Ren, Du, Stomach and Liver Channels • Kidney, uterus	Sea of Blood Sea of Twelve Channels	Disorders related to the Blood, irregular menstruation, infertility, miscarriage, dyspnea, abdominal cramps.
Dai	Circling the waist and abdomen	• Gall Bladder and Kidney Divergent Channel • Kidney, uterus	Bind and control all channels that run longitudinally.	Leukorrhea, paralysis, abdominal fullness and distention, pain of the lower back and legs
Yang Qiao	Lateral aspect of the lower extremities, hip, hypochondriac region, shoulder, neck, corner of the mouth, eye	• Urinary Bladder, Gall Bladder, Stomach, Large Intestine and Small Intestine Channels • Brain	Regulate the movement of and balance the Yang Qi of the left and right, medial and lateral sides of the lower extremities. Regulate the opening function of the eyes, normalize brain function.	Spasm of the lateral aspect of the lower extremities, epilepsy, insomnia, eversion of the foot
Yin Qiao	Medial aspect of the lower extremities, external genitalia, abdomen, stomach, and chest, supraclavicular fossa, throat, face, eye	• Kidney and Urinary Bladder Channels • Brain	Regulate the movement of and balance the Yin Qi of the left and right, medial and lateral sides of the lower extremities. Regulate the closing function of the eyes, normalize brain function.	Spasm of the medial aspect of the lower extremities, epilepsy, somnolence, inversion of the foot

Yang Wei	Lateral aspect of the lower extremities and abdomen, hypochondriac region, shoulder, retroauricular area, lateral side of the head	• Urinary Bladder, Gall Bladder, Stomach, Small Intestine, San Jiao, Large Intestine and Du Channels • None	Connect and regulate all the Yang Channels. Dominate the exterior.	Exterior syndromes, Shao Yang syndrome, disorders of the sides of the body.
Yin Wei	Medial aspect of the lower extremities, lower abdomen, stomach, hypochondriac region, diaphragm, chest throat, root of tongue	• Kidney, Spleen, Liver and Ren Channels • Interior organs	Connect and regulate all the Yin Channels. Dominate the interior	Interior disorders Stomach, heart, chest, and abdomen disorders

The Clinical Applications of the Eight Extraordinary Channels As They Are Traditionally Paired

There are eight points selected from the twelve channels called the *Opening Points*, one for each of the Eight Extraordinary Channels. There is a specific energetic link between the Opening Points and their related Eight Extraordinary Channels. The functions and indications of these eight points is expanded beyond the disorders of their own channel to include those of the Extraordinary Channel with which they are related. For example, SI 3 is used not only for disorders of the Small Intestine Channel, but also for the disorders of the Du Channel.

The Eight Extraordinary Channels are arranged in pairs. The Opening Point of each channel is used together with the Opening Point of its paired channel. When used in combination, these paired points affect disorders of specific areas of the body. Clinically, when one point is selected on the right side (e.g., Sp 4), its paired point (Pc 6) will usually be treated on the left side. Frequently, two pairs will be used together, further expanding the area of influence of the treatment, and creating an energetic circulation from left to right, and upward and downward, as symbolized in the Pa Gua (Eight Trigrams) and the Tai Ji (Yin/Yang symbol).

Opening and Paired Points of the Eight Extraordinary Channels

Channel	Opening and Paired Points	Treats Disorders of:
Du and Yang Qiao	SI 3/UB 62	Back, spine, neck, head, brain, eyes, posterior aspect of the legs
Ren and Yin Qiao	Lu 7/ Ki 6	Lung, chest, throat, abdomen, face
Chong and Yin Wei	Sp 4/Pc 6	Heart, stomach, chest, abdomen, medial aspect of the leg
Dai and Yang Wei	GB 41/SJ 5	Lateral aspect of the body, shoulders, neck and head, lateral aspect of the leg

Case Studies

The following twenty case studies demonstrate the clinical application of Channel Theory and the process of case analysis in the practice of acupuncture. The following symbols will be used to explain the treatment methods of each case.

Symbol	Treatment Method
⊥	Reducing
T	Reinforcing
I	Even
X	Moxa stick
Δ3	Small moxa cone. The number indicates how many cones.
Δ	Large moxa cone, with ginger, garlic, salt, or aconite in between
⇧	Warming needles
O	Cupping
⬇	Bleeding
Q	Intradermal needle
N	Electrical stimulation

Superscript letters designate whether a point is treated on the left (L), right (R), or both sides (B). For example, L UB 62 Δ5 indicates that the Urinary Bladder 62 was treated on the left side with five small moxa cones. R SI 11 ⊥ & O indicates that Small Intestine 11 was treated on the right side with reducing method followed by cupping.

Case 1   Costal Muscle Strain

Case History
A professional golfer, in his forties, complained of chest pain below the left nipple for ten days. The pain was sharp and spastic, referring to the lateral side of the chest, and the back beneath the inferior angle of the scapula. He also experienced a pulling sensation down the entire left side of his body. It was exacerbated by his golf swing as well as if he coughed, or breathed deeply. He often had to stop in mid-swing. Muscle relaxants had not provided him any relief.

Examination
Tongue:	Normal.
Pulse:	Slightly wiry.
Palpation:	Left side: There was a very tender spot at St 18, muscle spasm below the inferior angle of the scapula, muscle tightness on the lateral side of the hip and lower extremity. There was tenderness at UB 59 and UB 62.
	Right side: Tenderness at Lv 3.

Diagnosis
TCM:	Obstruction of Qi and Blood in the Urinary Bladder and Gall Bladder Tendinomuscular Channels and Collaterals.
WM:	Costal muscle strain.

Principle of Treatment
1) Activate Qi and Blood, remove obstruction in the channels and collaterals, loosen muscle spasms.

Prescription
Acupuncture
1) ^{L} UB 59 $^\perp$ ^{R} SI 6 $^\perp$

2) ^{L} Huatoujiaji (UB 15 level) $^{I\ \&\ O}$ ^{L} UB 58 $^\perp$ ^{R} GB 34 $^\perp$ ^{L} Pc 6 ^{I} Ashi points (*Hui Ci*[1] technique followed by cupping)

3) ^{L} St 18 $^\varphi$

Needles were inserted into the first group of points with the patient in a sitting position. He was asked to move the affected area by rotating his torso and left shoulder, and breathing deeply while the needles were manipulated. After fifteen minutes, the needles were removed and the second group of points were needled. At the completion of treatment, an intradermal needle was inserted at St 18.

Results
Fifteen minutes after the distal points were applied, eighty percent of the pain and spasm was relieved. At the end of the first treatment, the patient's pain was almost gone. The same prescription was repeated two days later, after which he patient was free of pain and able to compete in a golf tournament.

Analysis
This case applies the theory of the Urinary Bladder Tendinomuscular Channel and Yang Qiao Channel, and demonstrates the importance of careful channel differentiation. On first consideration, it would seem that the Stomach and Gall Bladder Channels were primarily involved in the chest pain. It should be noted, however, that the distribution of the Urinary Bladder Tendinomuscular Channel and Yang Qiao Channel also include the affected area. By doing a comprehensive palpation of the Urinary Bladder Channel, it was revealed that UB 58 and UB 59 were very tender and should be selected for treatment.

UB 59 and SI 6 are points of the Tai Yang Channels as well as the Xi (Cleft) points of the Yang Qiao and Small Intestine Channels respectively. When they are used contralaterally as the patient rotates the affected area, the Qi stagnation is quickly broken through and the pain alleviated. The Huatoujiaji point was selected to treat the lateral chest pain by stimulating the nerve root whose distribution enervates the area. The combination of UB 58, GB 34, and Pc 6 was used to open the channels and loosen the muscle spasms. Hui Ci technique was applied to the Ashi point, at the inferior angle of the scapula, to break through the muscle spasms. Retention of the intradermal needle on St 18 provided long term, gentle stimulation to prolong the treatment effect.

Case 2   Cervical Spine Injury

Case History
A male patient, age 45, had suffered from neck pain for six years. The pain had been caused by a work related injury in which he fell from a height, and landed on the crown of his head. The impact caused a compression fracture of the second and third cervical vertebrae, and a rupture of the disc between the fifth and sixth cervical vertebrae. He had undergone two surgeries during the first two years

---

[1] Refer to the description of the clinical applications of the Tendinomuscular Channels in chapter 1.

following the accident, but there had been minimal improvement of his pain. He was unable to perform any kind of physical activity which required him to turn his neck, and had been told he would have to live with the pain for the rest of his life. The thought that he might never improve caused him to be depressed. Although the patient had been in physical therapy since the first surgery, had been given numerous anti-inflammatory drugs and muscle relaxants, and had also tried chiropractic and acupuncture treatment, he had improved very little. His symptoms also included headache and neck stiffness upon awakening and restricted movement of the neck. The pain radiated to his right arm, and was accompanied by numbness in the hand, especially the ring and small fingers. He often experienced dizziness, chest discomfort, and lower back pain.

Examination

Tongue: Reddish purple with a white, sticky coating.
Pulse: Wiry, rolling, weak at the Chi regions.
Palpation: There was muscle strain and tightness, bilateral to the cervical vertebrae, a large nodule on the right side between GB 20 and GB 12. There were also muscle spasms and tenderness on the mediosuperior border of the right scapular spine, and bilaterally on the medial border of the scapula at the level of T 5 and T 6. There was a sensation of stagnation at SI 11, LI 15, and Jianneiling on the right side, tenderness at LI 10 and UB 23. The patient's cervical ranges of motion were restricted as follows: flexion - pain at 30°, extension - pain at 10°, left lateral flexion - pain at 30°, right lateral flexion - pain at 10°, left rotation - pain at 60°, right rotation - pain at 20°.

Diagnosis

TCM: Neck pain caused by traumatic injury resulting in obstruction of Qi and Blood in multiple
         channels and collaterals.
WM: Fracture of C2 and C3 with rupture of cervical disc between C5 and C6, muscular strain.

Principle of Treatment

1) Remove obstruction and activate circulation of Qi and Blood, stop pain and normalize the movement of the neck.
2) Promote the circulation, strengthen the tendons, ligaments, joints and bones, tonify the Liver and Kidney,

Prescription

Acupuncture

1)   Tapping with Seven Star Needles, Cupping and TDP lamp on the affected areas.

2) ^{R} SI 3 $\perp$ ^{L} Pc 6 $\perp$ Ren 24 $\perp$ Du 16 $\perp$

3) ^{R} UB 10 $^{\perp \& O}$ ^{R} GB 20 $^\perp$ ^{L} UB 62 $^\perp$ ^{R} UB 60 $^\perp$ ^{R} SI 11 $^{\perp \& O}$ ^{R} SI 12 $^{\perp \& O}$ ^{B} LI 10 $\perp$
     ^{B} GB 34 $^\perp$ ^{B} Lv 3 $^\perp$ ^{B} UB 23^T ^{L} Ki 4 ^{T} ^{R} GB 39 $^\perp$

Tapping with a Seven Star Needles was performed at a rate of 80 times per minute, along side the cervical and thoracic vertebrae (C1 - T 6), and on the nodules of the large muscles. This was immediately followed by cupping. This method is called ***Xu Ci Ba Guan***. A TDP lamp was applied afterwards.

The second group of points (except Du 16) was applied with the patient in sitting position. He was asked to flex, extend, and rotate the neck while the needles were manipulated. Needles were retained for 15 minutes, then Du 16 was added. Three or four points were selected from group three for each treatment, plus Ashi points with Hui Ci technique. The patient was given three treatments a week for four weeks, which was reduced to two visits a week for two months, then to one or two times per week for four months.

Case 3   Lupus Erythmatosis and Fibromyalgia (Bi Syndrome)

Case History

A female patient of 36, complained of muscle and joint pain, for several years. She had been diagnosed with lupus erythmatosis and fibromyalgia. She complained of pain accompanied by swelling, heaviness, and limited movement of all of the joints, but her lower back, knees, wrist, and nape, were primarily affected. The pain was exacerbated by over-exertion or emotional disturbances, but not especially influenced by weather changes. It actually improved when she had a cold or other infection. Other symptoms included chronic fatigue, loose stools, and scanty menstruation. Her complexion was sallow and pale. The patient had been treated unsuccessfully by steroidal and non-steroidal anti-inflammatory drugs, as well as immuno-suppressants.

Examination

Tongue: Pale with purplish spots on the sides, tender appearance, white coating, sticky and thick at the root.

Pulse: Thready and wiry in the left Guan region, forceless and weak in the Chi regions.

Palpation: There were many tender spots including UB 65, UB 62, SI 3, LI 11, LI 10, SJ 5, and Sp 6.

Diagnosis

TCM: Bi Syndrome due to long term accumulation of Wind Cold Damp, causing obstruction of Qi and Blood in the Channels and Collaterals, and Qi and Blood Deficiency.

WM: Lupus erythmatosis, fibromyalgia.

Principle of Treatment

1) Expel Wind Cold Damp, activate Qi and Blood circulation, remove obstruction from the Channels and Collaterals, tonify Qi and Blood.
2) Strengthen the Liver and Kidney, balance the immunity.

Prescription

Acupuncture

1) ^{L} UB 65 $^\perp$ ^{R} SI 3 $^\perp$ ^{B} Sp 21^I ^{B} Lv 8^I Yintang ^{I}

2)   Ren 9 $^{\perp X}$ Ren 7$^{\perp X}$ B St 25$^{\perp X}$ ^{B} St 36 ^{T}

3)   Du 3 $^{T\,\triangle 5}$ Du 4 $^{T\,\triangle 5}$ Du 14 $^{T O}$ ^{B} UB 11 $^{\perp O}$ ^{B} UB 52 ^{T}

Three groups of points were used in alternation with Ashi points added each time. The patient was treated twice a week for two months, then once a week for one month, then once a month after that. She has been in treatment for two years at the time of this writing, and is continuing to come for maintenance.

Herbs

Modifications of Xiao Huo Luo Dan (Minor Invigorate the Collaterals Special Pill), Xue Fu Zhu Yu Tang (Drive Out Stasis in the Mansion of Blood Decoction), and Gui Pi Tang (Restore the Spleen Decoction) were used.

Results

The swelling and pain of the joints and muscles were greatly reduced after one month of treatment, during which time the patient gradually stopped all her medication. At the end of the fourth month of treatment, her joint pain was almost completely gone and all other symptoms disappeared. At the time of this writing, the patient takes treatment once a month for maintenance and is taking herbs to strengthen the Liver and Kidney and for regulate the immunity.

Analysis

This case demonstrates the clinical application of the theory of the Ren, Du, and Urinary Bladder Channels. The patient's symptoms does not constitute a simple Bi Syndrome. This condition developed over the course of several years, due to the intermingling of Wind Cold Damp, obstruction of Qi and Blood in the Channels and Collaterals, and Deficiency of Qi, Blood, Liver, and Kidney. Because of the massive involvement of the joints, muscles, and channels, it is difficult for the practitioner to judiciously select only a few points. In order to avoid the "pincushion" effect, a complete understanding of channel theory is necessary.

The Urinary Bladder Channel dominates the disorders of the tendons and ligaments. For disorders of the spine and back UB 62 is ordinarily paired with SI 3, as the respective Confluent Points of Yang Qiao and Du Channels. In cases where there is massive involvement of muscles and joints, substituting UB 65, the Shu (Stream) point, is more effective.

Sp 21 is the Major Luo Collateral of the Spleen Channel, and therefore connects with all the Luo Collaterals. When combined with Lv 8, it is not only very effective for treating whole body pain, but also for nourishing and lubricating the tendons and muscles. Mild stimulation of Yintang calms the nervous system to alleviate pain. It also has the effect of regulating the autoimmune response, along with Du 14, Du 4, Ren 7, UB 11, and UB 52.

In the second and third prescriptions, the Ren and Du Channels are activated so that the circulation of Qi and Blood will naturally spread to all the other channels. UB 11 is the Influential point of the bones, and UB 52 stores the Essence. They are used in combination to tonify the Liver and Kidney, and nourish and strengthen the bones.

Case 4   Sciatica

Case History

A female patient, aged 38, limped into the office because of muscle spasms and burning pain in her left hip, which referred to the back of thigh. There was also numbness on the lateral side of her leg and on the dorsum and bottom of the foot. She had fallen a week ago while rollerblading. Her pain had been continuous since the accident and it had disturbed her sleep. Although she had been taking prescribed medication, she had gotten very little relief.

Examination

Tongue:	Normal color and body, with thick white coating on the root.
Pulse:	Wiry and choppy.
Palpation:	There was a muscle knot at GB 30, with tightness surrounding the area, tenderness at the Huatoujiaji point between L4 and L5 and at Yaoyan, UB 31, UB 39, UB 58, and Ki 4.

Diagnosis

<u>TCM:</u>   Qi and Blood obstruction in the Yang Qiao, Gall Bladder, and Urinary Bladder Channels.

<u>WM:</u>   Sciatica.

Principle of Treatment

1) Remove obstruction, activate circulation, and stop pain.

Prescription

Acupuncture

1)   ᴿ LI 4 ⊥   ᴸ UB 62 ⊥

2)   ᴿ SI 11 ⊥   ᴸ GB 30 ⊥ & O

LI 4 was punctured first until a strong Qi sensation was produced, then the patient was asked to walk around moving the hip joint for 10 minutes. The point was manually stimulated twice more during the treatment. UB 62 and the second prescription were added later. Treatment was applied once every other day.

Results

After the insertion of the needle at LI 4, the patient immediately felt a release of the muscle spasm, and a reduction of pain in her hip and leg. At completion of the first treatment, her burning pain was reduced by eighty percent, which lasted for one day. The same prescription was applied for five more treatments, which brought about the patient's complete recovery.

Analysis

This is an example of using the theory of the Yang Qiao Channel, and the Urinary Bladder and Gall Bladder Tendinomuscular Channels. The patient completely recovered in a few sessions with the use of only four points.

The entire radial aspect of the second metacarpal bone can be considered as part of the point LI 4, and is very effective for treating disorders of the whole body. This area is divided into three segments, the most distal of which is related to the Upper Jiao, the middle to the Middle Jiao, and the most proximal to the Lower Jiao. In this case, the Lower Jiao segment was chosen to address the acute muscle spasm of the hip. The contralateral point is most commonly used. UB 62 is used to open the Yang Qiao and Urinary Bladder Channels, and release muscle spasms. The contralateral combination of SI 11 and GB 30, breaks through stagnation and activates the circulation of both the Tai Yang and Shao Yang Channels.

Case 5   Shoulder and Cervical Arthritis, Irregular Menstruation

Case History

A female patient, aged 48, complained of shoulder pain and stiffness with restricted range of motion. She had suffered from these symptoms for one year. Upon examination the patient exhibited reduced circumduction of both shoulder joints, and reaching her arm behind her back was especially difficult. She also had pain on the left nape and scapular region, with numbness and tingling referring to the ring and small fingers. All of her symptoms were exacerbated by vigorous exercise of the upper body, such as rowing a boat, which was her favorite sport. She was thin, looked pale, complained of poor sleep, and her knees felt weak. Her menstruation had become progressively more scanty and her cycle prolonged.

Examination
Tongue: Swollen body, slightly pale and purple, with a sticky, white coating.
Pulse: Wiry, rolling, and forceless.
Palpation: There was a string-like muscle spasm along the medial scapular border on the left side, tenderness on SI 12, SJ 14, GB 21, and GB 20.

Diagnosis
TCM: Bi Syndrome caused by Wind Cold Damp, obstructing the channels and collaterals, resulting in stagnation of Qi and Blood, deficiency of Qi and Blood, Liver, and Kidney.
WM: Shoulder arthritis, cervicalgia, paravertebral myospasms, irregular menstruation.

Principle of Treatment
1) Eliminate Wind Cold Damp, activate circulation, remove obstruction, stop pain.
2) Tonify Qi and Blood, strengthen the Liver and Kidney, normalize menstruation.

Prescription
Acupuncture
1) ^{R} Sp 9 $^\perp$ ^{L} St 38 $^\perp$ ^{L} Lv 3 $^\perp$ ^{R} LI 10 $^\perp$ Gua Sha

2) ^{R} GB 34 ^{1} ^{L} Lv 3 ^{1} ^{L} SJ 5 $^\perp$ ^{R} Lu 7 ^{1} ^{L} Ki 6 ^{T} ^{B} Jiansanzhen⇑[1]

Sp 9 and St 38 were punctured first, after which Gua Sha method, with herbal oil and cupping were performed. Then the patient was asked to move and rotate both shoulders. The total procedure took fifteen minutes. The patient was then asked to lie down, and needles were inserted at Lv 3 and LI 10. The two prescriptions were used in alternation, two to three times per week.

Herbs
Gui Pi Wan (Restore the Spleen Pill), Feng Shi Xiao Tong Wan (Eliminate Wind Damp, Stop Pain Pill), Liu Wei Di Huang Wan (Six Ingredient Pill with Rehmannia) were used.

Results
After two treatments, her pain and restricted movement were substantially improved. After two months of treatment, her pain was completely gone, and the range of motion of her shoulders returned to normal. After taking herbal medicine for three months, her menstruation became regular.

Analysis
In this case, the patient's shoulder symptoms involved many channels. The treatment strategies used demonstrate the theory of the three Yang Tendinomuscular Channels of the Hand and the application of ***Miu Ci*** method *(treating the corresponding area of the opposite side)*.

According to the theory of Miu Ci method, Sp 11 or Sp 12 would ordinarily be selected to treat the shoulder symptoms. However, clinically speaking, Sp 9 is more commonly used. This point is especially effective when the Tai Yin and Tai Yang Channels are affected, and when reaching behind the back is restricted. St 38, treated ipsilaterally, is an empirical point for shoulder pain, and is especially effective when both the Yang Ming and Shao Yang Channels are affected. A key point of this treatment is having the patient rotate the affected joint while the needles are in place. The combination of LI 10 with Lv 3 balances the treatment by having one upper, one lower, one Yin, and one Yang point. Lv 3

---

[1] Jiansanzhen refers to one of two combinations of three needles on the shoulder: (1) LI 15, SJ 14, the point between SI 9 and 10. (2) LI 15, SJ 14 and Jianneiling. In this case the first group of points was used.

opens the free flow of Qi and LI 10 guides the flow of Qi to the upper body. LI 10 was also selected because the Large Intestine Tendinomuscular Channel knots on the shoulder and is largely distributed on the scapular region, nape, and spinal column.

The combination of GB 34 and Lv 3 is very effective for all types of Bi Syndrome. It promotes circulation, and relieves pain and stiffness in the muscles, tendons, ligaments, and joints. The combination of Lu 7 and SJ 5, treated contralaterally, activates circulation in the shoulders and arms. Jiansanzhen was treated with warming needles to expel the Wind Cold Damp and promote circulation in the shoulder. Lu 7 was used with Ki 6, Lv 3, and Sp 9 to tonify the Kidney, Liver, Qi, and Blood, and to regulate menstruation.

Case 6   Carpal Tunnel Syndrome

Case History

A women in her sixties suffered from tingling, numbness, and burning pain of both hands for many years. She had undergone two surgeries without relief and had been treated unsuccessfully with medication. The pain often woke her up at night. She was unable to use her hands much because of the pain, and her grip strength had become very weak. She also had lower back pain.

Examination

Tongue:	Tender, dark purplish with an uneven, white coating, sticky in some places.
Pulse:	Thready and weak on the right side, thready and wiry on the Guan region, weak on the Chi region on the left,
Palpation:	The muscles of both arms showed a general loss of tone. There were muscle spasms on the upper portion of m. brachioradialis, and lower portion of the m. deltoideus. There were surgical scars on the medial aspect of both wrists and tenderness at LI 11, LI 10, Lu 7, Pc 7, Pc 5, SI 4, and SJ 5.

Diagnosis

TCM:	Obstruction of Qi and Blood in the channels and collaterals of the arm, deficiency of Qi and Blood, underlying deficiency of the Kidney and Liver.
WM:	Carpal Tunnel Syndrome.

Principle of Treatment

1) Remove obstruction, promote circulation of Qi and Blood to the arms and wrists, alleviate pain.
2) Tonify the Qi, Blood, Kidney, and Liver.

Prescription
Acupuncture

1) ^{R} GB 34$^⊥$ ^{L} St 41$^⊥$ ^{R} SJ 5 - Pc 6 ^{R} Pc 5$^ |$ ^{R} LI 10$^{|\& ↑}$ ^{R} Pc 7$^{X \& Q}$

2) ^{B} UB 18^T ^{B} UB 23^T ^{B} UB 22^T ^{B} UB 25^T ^{L} Lu 7$^ |$ ^{R} LI 11$^{|\& ↑}$
   ^{R} SI 4$^ |$

After inserting needles in GB 34 and St 41, the patient was asked to rotate and tap her wrists and forearms with the opposite hand for ten minutes, then the rest of the needles were inserted. Threading method was used from SJ 5 to Pc 6.

The two groups of points were used in alternation twice a week. The patient was advised to do wrist exercises, tap her wrist joints, and do rubbing massage on her arms for ten minutes twice a day.

Herbs

Tian Qi Du Zhong Wan (Pseudoginseng and Eucommia Pill) and Su Jing Huo Xue Tang (Soothe the Tendons and Activate the Blood Decoction) were used.

Results

After the first treatment, the spastic, burning pain disappeared. At the end of the first course of ten treatments, the numbness and tingling were greatly reduced, and the patient began to regain sensation in her wrists. Treatment was continued for five months, during which her sensation and grip strength returned to normal. After completing treatment, she was able to perform her daily work without difficulty. Her lower back pain also greatly improved.

Analysis

This case demonstrates the application of Channel Theory to treat stubborn, painful disorders. The Pericardium, Large Intestine, and San Jiao Channels were mainly involved. There was a coexistence of both obstruction and deficiency of Qi and Blood in the channels. The combination of GB 34 and St 41 contralaterally was chosen for two reasons: 1) points below have an energetic influence on the areas above, in this case creating a relaxing effect on the tendons and ligaments of the wrist, and 2) inserting needles in the lower extremities rather than using local points allows the free movement of the wrist and arm during treatment.

SJ 5 threading to Pc 6, creates an energetic movement from the wrist and hand, up the arm. Pc 5 and LI 10 are local and adjacent points for wrist pain. Pc 7, with intradermal needle, gives a constant, mild stimulation to the affected area.

LI 11, with warming needle, together with Lu 7, promotes circulation in the whole arm. SI 4 is an empirical point for disorders of the wrist joint, as implied by its name Wangu (Wrist Bones). The Back Shu points were used to treat the underlying deficiency.

In my experience, gentle, manual needle stimulation or moxa offers more long lasting relief than using an electrical stimulator, which may cause after-sensations such as burning pain. In a case like this, daily exercise and massage is important to help open the channels, break up the stagnation, soften the scar tissue, and accelerate the healing process.

Case 7   Herpes Zoster (Toxic Damp Heat Syndrome)

Case History

A 20 year old woman complained of burning pain on her right hip which referred to the genital area. Her pain had begun one week before coming for treatment, and had been getting worse day by day. There were redness in the painful area as well as vessicles, several of which appeared to have turbid fluid in them. For the previous two days, she had noticed the same kind of pain in the area from the corner of her right eye to the temporal region. Her complexion was pale.

The patient's other symptoms included feverishness, disturbed sleep, irritability, restlessness, dry mouth, and dark, yellow urination. Her gynecological history included a recent vaginal infection, a history of genital herpes, and the fact that she had had several sexual partners. At the time, she was taking oral contraceptives.

Examination

Tongue: Pale with red, protruding spots in the area from the tip to the sides of the tongue. The coating was dirty, yellow, sticky, and dry.

Pulse:	Thready and slightly rapid, wiry, and rolling on both Guan regions.
Observation:	There were reddish lesions from UB 31 to GB 29, and to the inguinal groove on the right side, with a number of vessicles containing turbid fluid. There were similar lesions lateral to the right eye, but without fluid-filled vessicles.
Palpation:	There was tenderness on the Huatoujiaji points from L 2 to S 2, also at GB 26, GB 24, GB 41, GB 34, SJ 5, SJ 6, and GB 20.

Diagnosis

TCM:	Externally contracted toxic Damp Heat, stagnating in the Shao Yang, Dai, and Yang Wei Channels, consumption of Qi and Blood.
WM:	Herpes zoster.

Principle of Treatment

1) Eliminate toxic Damp Heat, remove channel obstruction, stop pain.
2) Regulate Qi and Blood.

Prescription

Acupuncture

1) ᴿ GB 1 ↓   ᴿ Longyanxue[1] ↓   ᴿ St 30 ↓   ᴸ GB 34 ⊥   ᴿ SJ 6 ⊥   ᴿ SJ 2 ⊥   Surrounding needles [2] ᴺ

2) ᴿ GB 41 ⊥   ᴸ SJ 5 ⊥   ᴿ GB 26 ⊥   ᴿ Sp 6 ⊥   ᴸ Sp 9 ⊥   ᴿ Pc 3 ⊥   ᴸ UB 40 ⊥

The first group of points was used for three treatments, then the two groups of points were used in alternation, three times per week for three weeks. Pricking method on GB 1 and St 30 was performed by pinching the skin before pricking the point, then squeezing out several drops of blood. Surrounding needles were used around the perimeter of the lesions, with transverse insertion, a maximum of five to ten degrees.

Herbs

Long Dan Xie Gan Wan (Gentiana Longdancao Pill to Drain the Liver Pill) was given for two weeks.

Results

The vessicles began shrinking after the first treatment and their color became much less red. The pain was also substantially reduced. A sterilized needle was used to open several of the fluid filled vessicles, after which the area was cleaned with betadine solution. Following the third treatment, the vessicles had all disappeared. Two weeks later, 90% of the pain and redness was gone, and at the end of the third week of treatment, the patient had completely recovered. She was advised to follow a more sanitary regimen of menstrual and sexual hygiene.

Analysis

This case demonstrates the successful use of the theory of the Shao Yang, Dai, and Yang Wei Channels. Because the patient was sexually active and had a history of herpes outbreaks, she easily contracted toxic Damp Heat. When Damp Heat stagnates in the Shao Yang, Dai, and Yang Wei Channels, it intermingles with and obstructs the Qi and Blood. This produces heat in the Blood, reddish skin lesions, vessicles, and severe pain along the channel's distribution.

---

[1] Longyanxue means *Point of the Eye of the Dragon*. It is located on the Small Intestine Channel on the small finger. Flex the finger, then take the point at the end of the skin crease on the lateral aspect at the junction of the first and second proximal phalanges.

[2] Shallow insertion at ten to fifteen degree angles of many needles around the affected area.

Pricking method at GB 1 and St 30 is very effective for quickly reducing toxic Damp Heat in the Blood. According to Traditional Chinese Medicine theory, the lesions of herpes zoster are called a *Fire Dragon*. Pricking method is applied to the *Eye of the Dragon* (Longyanxue) and the *Head of the Dragon* (in this case GB 1 and St 30). By "cutting off the dragon's head", further spreading and worsening of the lesions can be prevented.

GB 34, SJ 6, and SJ 2 clear Damp Heat and remove obstruction from the channels, on the sides of the body. An electrical stimulator was used on the Surrounding Needles along the border of the lesions to promote circulation and help dry up the vessicles.

In the second prescription, the combination of GB 41, SJ 5, and GB 26 open the Shao Yang, Yang Wei, and Dai Channels, and eliminate Damp Heat. Sp 6 and Sp 9 strengthen the Spleen and resolve Dampness. When Pc 3 is used in combination with UB 40 (which is the Xi (Cleft) point of Blood), they reduces fire toxin in the Blood.

Case 8   Rheumatoid and Osteoarthritis (Bi Syndrome)

Case History

A female patient in her fifties complained of swelling and pain of the joints for fifteen years. Her hands and feet were especially affected, and showed some deformity. She also complained of pain and stiffness of the nape, upper back, right shoulder, left hip, and lower back. Her pain was so often excruciating, that she suffered from depression, frustration, insomnia, and compulsive eating, which caused her to gain 30 lbs. during the last two years. She also had difficulty performing her duties as a secretary due to the pain. The symptoms were exacerbated by Cold Damp and stress. She had been taking numerous steroidal and non-steroidal anti-inflammatory drugs, including 800 mg. of Motrin 3-4 times per day, and 20 mg. of Prozac a day for depression. The medication provided only temporary relief.

Examination

Tongue: Swollen, dull, reddish purple, small cracks on the front, greasy and white coating.
Pulse: Deep, rolling, wiry and forceless.
Palpation: The lower extremities showed one degree of pitting edema, the knees were swollen and tender to the touch. The interphalangeal joints were swollen and deformed. There were numerous tender spots on many of the channels.

Diagnosis

TCM: Bi Syndrome due to contracted Damp Cold Wind intermingled with Phlegm resulting in stagnation of Qi and Blood in the joints and collaterals, underlying deficiency of Kidney,

Liver, and Spleen.
WM: Rheumatoid arthritis and osteoarthritis.

Principle of Treatment

1) Treating Biao and Ben simultaneously. Expel contracted Damp Cold Wind, activate circulation of Qi and Blood, remove stagnation, and stop pain.
2) Tonify and Kidney, Liver, and Spleen.

Prescription
Acupuncture
1)   ᴿ GB 39 ˈ   ᴿ GB 34⊥   ᴸ LI 4⊥   ᴸ LI 11 ˈ   ᴮ Sp 9 ˈ   Ren 5 ⇧

2) ^{B} UB 11 ^{I} ^{R} St 37 ^{I} ^{R} St 39 ^{I} ^{L} UB 65 ^{I} ^{L} Lv 8 ^{I} ^{L} Pc 6 ^{I} ^{R} LI 10 ^{I}

3) ^{L} UB 62 ^{I} ^{R} SI 3 ^{I} ^{B} UB 23 ^{TX} ^{B} UB 20 ^{TX} ^{B} Sp 6 ^{T} Cupping on the UB Channel
                                                          first line.

Treatment was given twice a week for two months, then reduced to once a week for a total of six months. Additional points such as Sp 6, St 36, LI 10, Sp 21, Baxie, and Neixiyan were used as modifications or local points. Seven Star Needles were used locally on the joints to reduce swelling and pain. An electrical stimulator and TDP lamp were sometimes used.

Herbs

The following patent formulas were used: Du Huo Ji Sheng Wan (Angelica Pubescens and Sangjisheng Pill), Shang Zhong Xia Tong Yong Tong Feng Wan (Pill for Pain Involving the Upper, Middle and Lower Jiao), Gu Zhi Zeng Sheng Pian (Bone Spur Pain Pill). An empirical formula designed by the author was given for the purpose of counter-acting the auto-immune response of the rheumatoid arthritis. The following herbs were included: Shu Di Huang (Rehmanniae Glutinosae Conquitae, Rx), Zao Jiao Ci (Gleditsiae Sinensis, Spina), Yin Yang Huo (Epimedii, Hb.), Gan Cao (Glycirrhizae Uralensis, Rx.), Hong Hua (Carthami Tinctorii, Fl.), and Du Huo (Angelica Pubescentis, Rx.).

Results

After the first two treatments, the patient felt fatigue and an aching over her whole body. She was unable to sleep at night. The same points were used for the succeeding treatments, but with gentle stimulation, and she began to improve. After two months of treatment, sixty percent of her pain was gone, the swelling and edema subsided. She was able to discontinued her Motrin and Prozac. After a total of six months of treatment, eighty percent of her symptoms were gone. The patient's acupuncture treatments were discontinued when she moved out-of-state, but she is still able to continue with the herbal prescriptions, which are shipped to her. At her two year follow-up, she is nearly symptom free and is able to work and live an active lifestyle.

Analysis

This case demonstrates the process of differential diagnosis for chronic and stubborn Bi Syndrome, when there are many channels involved. Damp Cold Wind was contracted in the channels and intermingled with Phlegm, which caused stagnation of Qi and Blood in the joints and collaterals. Due to the chronic nature of the disorder, Kidney, Liver, and Spleen became deficient. The channels which were mainly involved included the Gall Bladder, Urinary Bladder, Kidney, Stomach, and Large Intestine Channels.

The first prescription employs the theory, *Gall Bladder Channel dominates the disorders of the bones*, as stated in Chapter 10, "Chapter of Channels," Nei Jing, Ling Shu, (Spiritual Axis). The combination of GB 39 and GB 34, with LI 4 and LI 11, is effective for strengthening the bones and joints, removing obstruction, activating the Qi and Blood circulation, expelling contracted Cold Damp Wind, and reducing pain. Sp 9 strengthens the Middle Jiao, and resolves dampness. Ren 5 (Front Mu of San Jiao) addresses painful symptoms of the whole body.

The strategy of the second prescription is based on the principle, *to eliminate Wind treat the Blood first*. UB 11, St 37, and St 39 were selected because they are "Sea of Blood" points. When Blood is sufficient and circulating normally, there will be spontaneous elimination of contracted Damp Cold Wind. The combination of UB 65, the Shu (Stream) point, and Lv 8, the He (Sea) and Mother point, activates the Qi and Blood in the whole body, but especially in the lower extremities. Pc 6 calms the mind, relaxes the nerves, and stops pain. When it is used in combination with LI 10, the energetic influence covers not only the upper arm, but also the neck, nape, and upper back.

The third prescription is based on the theory that *Urinary Bladder Channel dominates the disorders of the tendons and ligaments*. UB 62 and SI 3 open the Urinary Bladder and Du Channels. When they are used with Sp 6, they nourish the Blood, tonify the Kidney and promote circulation in the

146

joints, tendons, ligaments, and bones. UB 23 and UB 20 are the Back Shu points of the Kidney and Spleen, and are used to tonify and their associated organs.

Cupping, moxibustion, electrical stimulation, warming method, and Seven Star Needles played an important role in breaking up the deeply rooted stagnation. Herbal prescription was also vital for treatment of both Biao and Ben, especially for the underlying deficiency and auto-immune disease. When the patient relocated to a dryer climate, she maintained her improvement without acupuncture, further demonstrating the importance of treating Dampness in her case.

Case 9   Ulcerative Colitis, Asthma

Case History
A female patient, age 43 was diagnosed with ulcerative colitis five years ago. Her chief complaint was mucus and blood in the stool, accompanied by lower abdominal cramping and pain. These symptoms were exacerbated by poor diet and emotional distress. She also suffered from chronic asthma, allergies, often felt short of breath, had stiffness and pain in her upper back and shoulder, and soreness of the lower back. She had been treated with a number of steroidal and non-steroidal anti-inflammatory drugs with little effect.

Examination

Tongue: Dull, reddish purple with teeth marks, small cracks on the surface, and a white and sticky coating. The tongue body was tender and puffy in the Lung area.

Pulse: Deep, thready, and wiry. The Lung pulse extended to the thenar eminence. Both Chi regions were weak.

Palpation: There was a sense of stagnation at St 25 and St 37 bilaterally[1], tenderness at Du 12, UB 44, UB 30, and UB 57. There was a soft and empty feeling at Ren 6, muscle strain and tightness at UB 13, a nodule and tenderness at Lu 6, and several tender points along the Large Intestine Channel. The lower left abdomen was tender in the area from GB 29 to Sp 13.

Diagnosis
TCM: Qi, Blood, and Damp Heat stagnating in the Large Intestine, Phlegm accumulation in the Lung, Lung and Kidney Qi Deficiency.

WM: Ulcerative sigmoid colitis, allergic asthma.

Principle of Treatment
1) Remove stagnation of Qi and Blood, resolve and clear Damp Heat, regulate the function of Large Intestine, harmonize the Lung and Large Intestine.
2) Tonify Lung and Kidney Qi, resolve phlegm, promote circulation in the Lung and the Large Intestine.

Prescription
Acupuncture
1) ^{R} Lu 6 $^\perp$ ^{L} St 37 $^|$ ^{R} St 25 $^\perp$ Du 12 $^|$ ^{B} UB 30 ↑

2) ^{B} UB 13 $^{|\&O}$ Du 3 ↑ ^{B} UB 25 $^|$ ^{B} St 36 ^{T} ^{L} Pc 6 $^|$ Ren 6 ^{T}

---

[1] A feeling of hardness, thickness, a temperature variation from the are adjacent to the point being palpated or some combination of these qualities. Such points are also usually tender to the touch.

The first prescription was used twice a week for ten treatments, during the course of which it was modified by adding or rotating in Ren 6 with Ren 17, St 36, Sp 6, and UB 25. The second prescription was applied for an additional thirty treatments over the following six months. Points used in addition, and rotation in included UB 44, Sp 15, Lv 3, Sp 9, UB 20, and UB 23. The patient experienced two mild asthmatic attacks during the course of treatment. At those times, only the following points were used: Lu 6, Ren 17, Dingchuan, SI 11, St 40, Pc 6, and Lu 7.

Herbs

Liu Jun Zi Tang (Six Gentlemen) and Shen Ling Bai Zhu San (Codonopsis, Poria and Atractylodes Powder) were used as base formulas. They were modified by adding herbs from the invigorate blood, tonify blood, and stop bleeding categories, such as raw Shen San Qi (Rx. Pseudoginseng), Huai Hua (Flos Sophorae), Di Yu (Rx. Sanguisorbae), and Dang Gui (Rx. Angelica sinensis).

Results

After the first course with the first prescription, the mucus and blood in the patient's stool was completely gone. Her lower abdominal pain and cramping were reduced to a slight discomfort. Over the course of the next thirty treatments, all her asthmatic and allergic symptoms steadily decreased. During this time, there were only two mild asthmatic attacks, which were induced by exposure to pollen and dust. The patient was released from treatment, symptom free. Two years later, she has maintained her health, and continues to come for monthly balancing treatments.

Analysis

This case demonstrates the successful application of the theory of the Lung and Large Intestine Channels. This patient had chronic, allergic asthma, and a congenital deficiency of Lung Qi which was indicated by the extended Lung Pulse. Over the years, the function of the Large Intestine, was disturbed which allowed the accumulation of Damp Heat, and stagnation of Qi and Blood in the Large Intestine. This caused chronic blood and mucus in the stool to develop. This is demonstrative of the process by which the pathological development of a disorder passes from one channel to another, due to their interconnection.

The treatment strategy was initially focused on two goals: 1) regulating the function of the Large Intestine and, 2) harmonizing the Lung and Large Intestine. In this case, treatment of the Spleen and Stomach had to be considered because of their interrelationship with the Lung and Large Intestine.

Lu 6 was selected as the chief point, not only because it is the Xi (Cleft) point of the Lung, but also due to its energetic influence on the anus and sigmoid colon. The combination of Du 12 and Lu 6 is very effective for treating simultaneous disorders of the Lung and Large Intestine. St 37 and St 25, the Lower He (Sea) point and Front Mu point of the Large Intestine Channel, have a direct effect on the large intestine organ. UB 30 was treated with a warming needle to promote circulation in the Lower Jiao.

The second prescription focused on strengthening the Lung, Large Intestine, and Kidney. For this purpose, UB 13 and UB 25, the Back Shu points of the Lung and Large Intestine Channels, were selected, and used in combination with Du 3. Ren 6, St 36, and Pc 6 were employed to enhance the immunity, resolve phlegm, and decrease the patient's sensitivity to allergens. UB 20 and UB 23, the Back Shu points of the Spleen and Kidney, were used for tonifying Spleen and Kidney Qi. The muscle spasm and strain at UB 13 was released by inserting two needles, pointed obliquely toward each other, one from above and one from below. Cupping was applied immediately after removing the needles. The patient was advised to do breathing exercises, Tai Ji Quan, and maintain a good diet.

Case 10   Aphonia, Depression (Plum Pit Qi Syndrome)

Case History

A female flight attendant, 37 years old, suddenly lost her voice two weeks before coming for treatment. She also complained of a chronic sensation, as if a foreign body was lodged in her throat. She was in the process of getting a divorce, and frequently experienced a variety of emotional symptoms including anxiety, depression, anger, sadness, weeping, and grief. She often felt like she could not catch her breath, had alternating diarrhea and constipation, and suffered from dream-disturbed sleep. She had lost weight, which she attributed to having a poor appetite. Other signs and symptoms included dark circles under the eyes, holding her shoulders in a hunched position, pain and stiffness of the shoulder joints, and tightness and pain on the bilaterally on m. tibialis.

Examination

Tongue: Red tip, pale and purple sides, with a thin, yellow, sticky, and dry coating.
Pulse: Thready, wiry, and choppy.
Palpation: The muscles around the shoulder and neck were tight. There was a ropy muscle spasm along the spine of the upper and middle back, and tenderness at LI 6, LI 11, LI 15, SI 11, SI 15, Lv 3, Sp 6, and St 40.

Diagnosis

TCM: Disharmony between Wood and Earth, stagnation of Liver Qi resulting in accumulation of Phlegm and Qi in the throat (Plum Pit Qi).

WM: Aphonia, chronic pharyngitis, anxiety, and depression.

Principle of Treatment

1) Soothe and smooth the Liver Qi, resolve Phlegm, harmonize Wood and Earth.
2) Nourish the Liver Yin and Blood, regulate the Liver Qi.

Prescription

Acupuncture

1) ^{L}Lv 3 $^|$ ^{L}Lv 2 $^\perp$ ^{R}LI 4 $^|$ ^{R}LI 3 $^\perp$ ^{L}Ht 5 $^|$ ^{R}St 40 $^\perp$ Ren 23 $^|$

2) ^{L}Lv 3 $^|$ ^{R}GB 34 $^|$ ^{L}Ki 6 ^{T} ^{R}Lu 7 ^{B}St 36 ^{T} ^{B}Liyan $^|$ (1 cun anterior to SI 17)

The first prescription was used three times per week for one week, then reduced to two times per week for an additional two weeks. The patient was then advised to take a one week break, after which treatments resumed with the second prescription, once per week for another four treatments.

Herbs

Modifications of Xiao Yao San (Rambling Powder) and Ban Xia Hou Po Tang (Pinellia and Magnolia Bark Decoction) were given as herbal powder formulas.

Results

After three sessions, the patient regained her voice, the foreign body sensation in her throat was greatly reduced, and her emotional symptoms were also significantly improved. An additional four treatments were given, after which her symptoms, including the muscle pain and tightness, were completely gone. Her physical and emotional condition became stable after completing the second course of treatment. Since her divorce had not been finalized, and she would be under continuing emotional strain, the patient was advised to take maintenance treatments every two week until the situation was resolved.

Analysis

This case is an example of applying the theory of the Liver Channel, and of Stomach and Heart Luo Collaterals. The patient's loss of voice and Plum Pit Qi symptoms were both due to emotional distress over her divorce. The pathogenesis of this patient was Liver Qi stagnation. When Liver Qi was stagnant, it caused 1) stagnation of Heart Qi, resulting in anxiety, depression, and dream-disturbed sleep, 2) Disharmony between Liver and Spleen, resulting in poor appetite, and diarrhea and constipation alternately, 3) accumulation of Phlegm and Qi in the throat (as the Liver Channel passes through the throat and nasopharynx).

The tightness and spasm of the muscles around the shoulder, neck, back, and m. tibialis were due to restrained Liver Qi, causing nervous tension and failure of Liver Blood to nourish the muscles, ligaments, and tendons.

The first prescription contains the combination Lv 2 and Lv 3 with LI 3 and LI 4. It is collectively known as ***Double Four Gates***. When these pairs of points are used contralaterally, they have a powerful effect in breaking through stagnation of Liver Qi, and promoting the free flow of Qi throughout the body. In my experience, this combination is very effective for many emotional disorders.

The Luo Collaterals of the Heart and Stomach Channels connect with the throat and vocal cords. When Ht 5 and St 40 are used together, they remove stagnation in this area and resolve the accumulation of Phlegm and Qi.

Long term stagnation of Liver Qi will ultimately cause consumption of Blood and Yin. The second prescription uses the combination of Ki 6 and Lu 7, Lv 3, St 36, and GB 34 to nourish the Blood and Yin, promote the circulation, relax the muscles, and lubricate the ligaments, tendons, and joints.

Case 11   Neurasthenia (Dizziness and Vertigo)

Case History

A male patient, aged 36, had suffered from frequent attacks of dizziness and vertigo for four weeks. He also experienced nausea, blurring of vision, photophobia, palpitations, sweating, and difficulty breathing. Occasionally, he had numbness and tingling running from his neck to his lower extremities. For two days he had had a constant headache, which he described as muscle strain, and a pulling sensation from the GB 19 area to the vertex, and to the UB 2 area. He also suffered from depression, anxiety, insomnia, and was afraid of going to work. A neurologist and an ENT specialist were consulted without a conclusive diagnosis. During their examinations, his physicians always recorded a high blood pressure. When taken at home or in my office, his blood pressure was never high. The patient's family medical history indicated a strong tendency toward diabetes, but his blood chemistry, including glucose tolerance test, was normal. He was a vegetarian.

Examination

Tongue: Slightly pale with teeth marks on the edges of the tongue.
Pulse: Thready, rapid, and choppy. Weak, with deep pressure, on the right Guan region.
Palpation: The patient's stomach was tight with a large spasmed area. His hands and feet were cold and clammy. There was a muscle spasm on the right side of his neck at the GB 19 area, and tenderness at UB 2 and Du 20. Pressure on Du 20 felt good to him.

Diagnosis

TCM: Dizziness and vertigo, upward disturbance of Liver Wind due to Liver Qi Stagnation and Liver Blood Deficiency, Disharmony between Wood and Fire.
WM: Neurasthenia.

Principle of Treatment

1) Treat **Ben** by tonifying the Blood, nourish the Liver, and smooth Liver Qi. The **Biao** (Liver Wind) will naturally be extinguished, and Wood and Fire will be harmonized.

Prescription

Acupuncture

1) ^{L} SJ 3 $^|$ Du 20 $^{|\&x}$ Ren 12 $^|$ ^{R} Lv 3 $^\perp$

2) ^{B} UB 18 ^{T} ^{B} UB 20 ^{T} ^{L} Pc 6 $^|$ ^{R} Sp 6 ^{T} ^{B} GB 20 $^|$

3) Ear acupuncture: Shenmen   Brain   Liver   Stomach   Heart

The patient was treated twice a week with the first group of points for two weeks, then with the second group for four weeks. Two or three ear points were selected each time, and embedding needles were inserted.

Herbs

Bu Zhong Yi Qi Wan (Tonify the Middle and Augment the Qi Pill), Gan Mai Da Zao Wan (Licorice, Wheat, and Dates Pill), Xiao Yao Wan (Rambling Pill) were used in alternation.

Results

After the first treatment, the patient's symptoms completely disappeared for two days. At his second treatment, he reported that while he was at his doctor's office, his blood pressure was checked three times over the course of several hours. The readings were in the range of 160 to 150 mm Hg systolic, and 100 to 108 mm Hg diastolic. He was nervous and frightened, then all his symptoms came back. After the second treatment, his symptoms again disappeared. He was given a few more treatments, twice weekly with the first prescription, and his condition remained stable.

The second group of points were used twice a week for four weeks, during which his pulse and tongue became completely normal. His symptoms disappeared and did not return. At a six month follow-up he was still completely symptom free.

Analysis

This case involves the clinical application of the theory of the Liver Channel, San Jiao Divergent Channel, and Du Channel. The patient's dizziness and vertigo were due to Liver Qi Stagnation and Liver Blood Deficiency, which caused an upward disturbance of Liver Wind. In this instance, by treating the *Ben* the *Biao* will naturally be treated as well. In other words, by tonifying Liver Blood, smoothing Liver Qi, and Lift the Spirit, Liver Wind will be extinguished.

In first prescription, the combination of Lv 3, SJ 3, and Du 20 with moxa is very effective for tonifying Liver Blood, and Lifting the Spirit. Note that Du 20 is the point where the San Jiao Divergent Channel begins and the Liver Channel ends. Ren 12 tonifies the source of Qi and Blood. In this case, it was used to consolidate and ground the Qi in the Middle Jiao.

In the second prescription, UB 18 and UB 20 tonify and strengthen the Liver and Spleen, while Sp 6 and Pc 6 harmonize Wood and Fire. GB 20 extinguishes Liver Wind. The ear acupuncture points were used to strengthen and continue the effect of the treatment.

Case 12   Hyperthyroidism (Phlegm Fire Obstructing the Liver and Heart)

Case History

A female patient, aged 37, came for treatment with multiple complaints. She suffered from fatigue, mood swings, tremors of the hands, palpitations, sweating, shortness of breath, dry mouth, bad breath, and alternating constipation and diarrhea. She had tightness and spasms of the stomach, which sometimes made her unable to each. Consequently, she had lost a significant amount of weight. Her facial complexion was dark and lusterless. Two years ago, she had been diagnosed with hyperthyroidism. Since then, her symptoms had been progressively worsening, and her physician had recommended radioactive iodine (I-131) treatment.

Examination

Tongue: Red spots at the tip, pale with many purplish spots on both edges of the tongue. Thin, sticky, and yellowish coating.

Pulse: Thready, rapid, and forceless.

Palpation: Muscle spasms in the epigastrium, tenderness and tightness from the right hypochondriac
region down to the lower abdomen. There were many tender points, including LI 4, St 43, Sp 6, St 36, and UB 22. Muscle spasms could also be palpated at UB 17, UB 10, and UB 52. Her thyroid was slightly enlarged.

Diagnosis

TCM: Long term stagnation of Qi and Blood, turning into Excessive Fire, intermingled with Phlegm, which further consumes Yin and weakens the Middle Jiao, Disharmony between Wood and Earth, obstruction of the San Jiao, Liver, and Heart Channels.

WM: Hyperthyroidism.

152

Principle of Treatment

1) Clear Fire, resolve Phlegm, regulate Qi and Blood, remove stagnation from the San Jiao, Liver and Heart Channels.
2) Tonify Yin, harmonize and strengthen the Middle Jiao.

Prescription

Acupuncture

1)	^{R} SJ 4 $^{\text{I or }\Delta 3-5}$	Ren 12 ^{I}	^{L} Lv 3 $^\perp$	^{L} Pc 6 ^{I}	^{R} St 40 $^\perp$	^{B} UB 10 ^{I}
2)	^{R} SJ 5 $^\perp$	^{L} St 43 (2) $^\perp$	^{L} Pc 5 ^{I}	^{B} St 36 ^{T}	^{L} Ht 3 $^\perp$	^{B} Ki 6 ^{T}
3)	^{B} UB 22 ^{T}	^{B} UB 17 ^{T}	^{B} UB 11 ^{I}	^{B} UB 52 ^{T}	^{L} Ki 9 ^{I}	^{R} LI 11 $^\perp$

Each group of points was used for five to ten treatments, two sessions per week, then the next group was substituted. This regimen was used for four months, after which the frequency of treatment was reduced gradually to once per week or every other week. The complete course of treatment was one year.

Herbs

Modifications of Yi Guan Jian (Linking Decoction), Ba Zhen Tang (Eight Treasures Decoction), Shen Mai Yin (Generate the Pulse Pill), and Xue Fu Zhu Yu Tang (Remove Stasis from the Mansion of Blood Decoction) were used.

Results

The patient improved with each treatment. After four months, most of her symptoms were gone, but her thyroid was still somewhat swollen. After one year of treatment, the swelling was gone, her thyroid tests were normal, and her medical doctor told her she no longer had hyperthyroidism.

Analysis

This is a complicated condition involving stagnation of Blood, Fire, and Phlegm, and deficiency of Yin, Qi, and Blood in many organs and channels. The Stomach, Kidney, Liver, and San Jiao Channels were especially affected.

According to Channel Theory, the San Jiao Channel dominates the disorders of Qi. It also regulates the function of the lymphatic and endocrine systems. When Qi in the San Jiao Channel is activated, the stagnation of pathogenic factors in all the other channels will naturally be removed.

The combination of SJ 4, Ren 12 and Lv 3 is very effective for the disorders of the endocrine system, especially hyperthyroidism and hypothyroidism. This is an example of treating the root cause of the disease, i.e. *Ben* treatment, rather than selecting numerous points to treat the myriad of symptoms. Clinically, it is always advisable to limit the number of needles used to avoid the "traffic-jam" of Qi effect.

The combinations of St 40 with Pc 6, and St 36 with Pc 5, are for regulating Qi and dissolving Phlegm. SJ 5 with St 43(2) [1], helps circulate Qi to the thyroid, especially when the Shao Yang and Yang Ming Channels are simultaneously disordered. Ht 3 and Ki 6 tonify the Yin and clear Heart Fire. UB 10 is an adjacent point for the thyroid area.

The Back Shu points in the third group were used to tonify all the related organs. Ki 9 is the Xi (Cleft) point of the Yin Wei Channel, and is very effective for detoxification when pathogenic factors are deeply rooted in the body. When it is combined with LI 11, the treatment effect is focused on the thyroid gland, to clear heat toxin and promote circulation.

---

[1] St 43 (2) indicates the point lateral to St 43. It is located in the depression distal to the junction of the third and fourth metatarsal bones.

Case 13　　Nervous Stomach, Irritable Bowel Syndrome

Case History

A male attorney, aged 54, complained of tightness and discomfort of the whole abdomen for eight to ten years. He frequently suffered attacks of intense spasm and pain, and had been admitted to the hospital several times due to severe attacks. His medical exams revealed a mild case of gastritis and irritable bowel syndrome. Other symptoms included nervous tension, hunger with no desire to eat, cramps below the heart area, alternating diarrhea and constipation, restlessness, poor sleep, fatigue, dry mouth, repeated outbreaks of oral herpes, a dark and dull complexion, and lower back pain.

Examination

Tongue:　　Dark, dull, reddish purple, swollen, dry with many small cracks. A thin, white, and dirty coating, thick at the middle and the root.

Pulse:　　Deep, tight, wiry, and thready. Weak at the right Guan and left Chi regions.

Palpation:　　The entire stomach area was tight. A muscle knot was felt on the left side of the stomach area. There was tenderness at Ren 10, Ren 9, St 24, Sp 14, Lv 13, and Ki 16. There were muscle spasms along the left side of the spine from T5 to L1. There was a feeling of softness and emptiness at the level of L 2 and L 3.

Diagnosis

TCM:　　Stagnation of Qi and Blood in the Middle Jiao, Disharmony between the Liver and Stomach, Qi and Yin Deficiency of the Kidney and Spleen.

WM:　　Nervous stomach, irritable bowel syndrome,.

Principle of Treatment

1) Regulate and strengthen the Qi in the Middle Jiao, harmonize the Liver and Stomach
2) Tonify Kidney, strengthen the Spleen.

Prescription

Acupuncture

1)　ᴸ Pc 6 ⁱ　　ᴿ Sp 6 ᵀ　　Ren 10 ⁱ　ᴸ Lv 14 ⊥　ᴿ St 25 ⊥　ᴸ Gua Sha UB 17 - 22 ⁸ᴼ

2)　ᴸ Ki 6 ᵀ　　ᴿ Lu 7 ⁱ　　ᴸ Ki 9 ᵀ　ᴮ Ki 16 ⁱ　　Ren 12 ⁱ　　ᴮ St 36 ᵀ

3)　ᴸ UB 17 ᵀ⁸ᴼ　ᴸ UB 19 ᵀ⁸ᴼ　Du 12 ⁱ　ᴸ UB 20 ᵀ ᵒʳ ↑　ᴮ UB 23 ᵀ ᵒʳ ↑　ᴮ UB 57 ⁱ

Treatment was given twice a week for one month, then once a week for another three months. Each of the three groups of points was used in rotation for five to ten sessions. After each treatment, one to three intradermal needles were put into the tender spots of the abdomen.

Herbs

Modifications of Si Ni San (Frigid Extremities Powder), Wu Mo Yin Zi (Five Milled-Herb Decoction), Shao Yao Gan Cao Tang (Peony and Licorice Decoction), and Sheng Mai San (Generate the Pulse Powder) in the form of herbal powders were administered. The dosage was three grams, three times a day.

Results

After the first two sessions, the patient was pleased to find himself free of pain for one whole day. After ten sessions, he could go for five to seven days without much discomfort. Altogether, he was treated for four months and, except for two mild occurrences when he was required to appear in court, he was able to maintain a stable condition. At the time of this writing, he has been symptom free for one

154

year, and continues to come once a month for maintenance treatments. These consist primarily of intradermal needles on Ren 12 and Sp 15.

Analysis

This case demonstrates the application of the theory of the Kidney, Spleen/Stomach, and Liver Channels. Initially, it seemed that the stress of his occupation caused the tightness and discomfort in his stomach. Due to the chronic nature of his illness, Kidney Deficiency had also developed. The patient had many symptoms which, according to Channel Theory, indicated the involvement of the Kidney, such as hunger without desire to eat, dark complexion, lower back pain, and a knotted feeling below the heart (the Kidney Luo Collateral goes to the area below the heart). The treatment strategy was divided into two steps:

1) *Break through the stagnation and release the muscle spasms.* For this purpose, Pc 6 and Sp 6 were used to ease nervous tension, release muscle spasms, and harmonize the Liver, Stomach, and Spleen. When Lv 14, Ren 10, and St 25 are used in combination, they form a diagonal line across the abdomen which, in my experience, has a powerful effect in breaking up stagnation in that area. Gua Sha method is applied immediately, followed by cupping, which is very effective for promoting circulation, releasing muscle spasms, and assisting the acupuncture in regulating the Qi. Intradermal needles were used on tender spots for continued gentle stimulation and relaxing the muscles.

2) *Strengthen and tonify the Spleen and Kidney.* This was mainly accomplished with the second and third prescriptions. Ki 6 and Lu 7 are Influential points, which tonify Kidney and regulate the Middle Jiao. The combination of UB 17 and UB 19 (known as the Four Flowers) is effective for tonifying Qi and Blood. The Back Shu points of the Spleen and Kidney Channels were used to warm up and tonify the Kidney and Spleen Yang, dispel internal Cold, and release spasms. The combination of Ki 9 and Ki 16 was used to tonify the Kidney and detoxify deeply root stagnation in the Middle Jiao. UB 57 is a special point for "opening the appetite," and promoting digestion and absorption as described in *Entrance of Medicine* by Li Yan of the Ming Dynasty. In my experience, Du 12 is not only promotes and tonifies Lung Qi, but is also effective for tonifying the large intestine, and normalizing the bowel movements.

Case 14   Ovarian Cyst

Case History

A female patient, aged 25, suffered from cramping and pain on the right side of the abdomen for five months. Her symptoms were worse during ovulation and before menstruation. There was swelling and distention in the painful area, which sometimes referred to the groin or hypochondriac region. Other symptoms included occipital headache and stiffness of the neck, increased volume of white, odorless vaginal discharge, and a pulling sensation and discomfort on her entire right side, including tightness of the TMJ, and medial aspect of the thigh. Her medical exam revealed an ovarian cyst, 6 x 7 cm on the right side. She had been using a sub-dermal, time-release estrogen implant as her contraceptive method for one year prior to developing these symptoms.

Examination

Tongue: Swollen tongue body, normal color. Striated, sticky coating at the root.
Pulse: Generally normal, but becoming wiry, rolling, and forceful during episodes of pain.
Palpation: Swelling and tenderness in the right lower abdomen, tenderness at St 28, GB 28, Kidney Essence point, Lv 9, UB 10, and UB 32.

Diagnosis

<u>TCM:</u>   Congealed Qi, Blood, Dampness, and Phlegm in the Ren and Chong Channels, dysfunction of the Kidney and Liver.

<u>WM:</u>   Ovarian Cyst, 6 x 7 cm on the right side.

Principle of Treatment

1) Activate the circulation of Qi and Blood in the Ren and Chong Channels, resolve phlegm and dampness, dissolve cysts.

2) Normalize the function of the Kidney and Liver.

Prescription

Acupuncture

1) ^{B} UB 11 $^⊥$ ^{R} St 37 $^⊥$ ^{L} St 39 $^⊥$ ^{B} Lv 5 $^⊥$ ^{R} UB 32 $^{X \& Q}$ Ren 3 ^{I}

2) ^{L} Sp 4 ^{I} ^{R} Pc 6 ^{I} ^{R} GB 26 $^⊥$ ^{R} GB 41 $^{⊥ \& N}$ ^{L} SJ 5 $^{⊥ \& N}$ ^{R} St 28 $^{⊥ \& N}$ ^{L} St 30 $^{⊥ \& N}$ ^{B} Kidney Essence pt. $^{Δ5 \& Q}$

Acupuncture was applied once every other day, from the seventh to the sixteenth day of her menstrual cycle, and from the seventh day preceding menstruation, through the second day of menstruation, a total of eight to ten treatments monthly. The two groups of points were used in alternation.

Herbs

Modifications of Gui Zhi Fu Ling Wan (Cinnamon Twig and Poria Pill) and Shao Fu Zhu Yu Tang (Drive Out Stasis in the Lower Abdomen), in the form of herbal powders were administered. The dosage was three grams, three times a day. Herbal powders were taken for the five days before menstruation, and five days around ovulation.

Results

After one month of treatment, the cramping and pain was greatly reduced. At the end of the second month of treatment, the puffiness and swelling of the lower abdomen disappeared. After the third month of treatment, the ovarian cyst was completely gone, confirmed by ultrasound.

Analysis

This case demonstrates the application of Liver, Kidney, Chong, and Ren Channel theory. This young woman's ovarian cyst was due to an hormonal imbalance, related to contraceptive use. In Traditional Chinese Medicine theory, this kind of imbalance usually involves a dysfunction of the Liver and Kidney, and stagnation of the Chong and Ren Channels. Nodules and cysts are often the result of congealed Qi, Blood, Dampness, and Phlegm.

UB 11, St 37, and St 39, the "Sea of Blood" points, are commonly used in gynecological disorders. In this case, they activate blood circulation, regulate the hormones, and dissolve cysts. Lv 5, the Luo (Connecting) point of the Liver Channel, is used together with UB 32 and Ren 3, for promoting circulation, and opening blockages in the Ren Channel and the pelvic region.

Sp 4 and Pc 6 are Influential points, which open the Chong Channels and remove stagnation. GB 41 and SJ 5 (treated by electrical stimulator), and GB 26, are effective for breaking through stagnation on the lateral aspect of the body, and in this case, especially target the abdomen. St 28 and St 30, treated contralaterally with electrical stimulator, are used as local points to break up congestion. The Kidney Essence point, with intradermal needles and moxa, is effective for activating circulation in the Lower Jiao and normalizing the function of the Kidney.

Case 15   Headache, Chronic Gastritis

Case History
A middle aged man suffered from frontal headaches, and pain and distention in the epigastrium for several years. He had taken Tagamet for months at a time, but it provided only temporary relief. Stress, eating chocolate, sweets, or MSG, often precipitated his headaches, which would usually be accompanied by nausea, vomiting, and diarrhea. He was a smoker, and often felt a stickiness in his mouth. Occasionally, he complained of tension and back pain.

Examination
Tongue: Flabby and swollen, dark and dull red with a thick, light yellow coating.
Pulse: Wiry and weak in the right Guan position with deep pressure.
Palpation: Tightness in the center of the epigastrium, tenderness at Ren 13, Ren 10, GB 24, St 25, St 37, Sp 6, and St 43. Muscle spasms were palpated on the back from the level of T 9 to L 2.

Diagnosis
TCM: Yang Ming headache due to upward disturbance of turbid Qi, and Dampness. Stomach pain due to obstruction of Qi and Damp Heat in the Middle Jiao,
WM: Headache, chronic gastritis.

Principle of Treatment
1) Clear Damp Heat, remove obstruction, regulate Stomach Qi, and stop the headache.
2) Harmonize and strengthen the Middle Jiao.

Prescription
Acupuncture

1)	B St 30	L St 37 ⊥	R LI 11⊥	B Sp 6 T	Ren 10	Yintang
2)	R Sp 4	R Sp 5	L Pc 6	L Pc 5	B St 8	B St 43 T
3)	Ren 12	B UB 20 T	B UB 21 T	B UB 17 T	B GB 30 ⊥	B St 36 T

Prescriptions one and two were used alternately, two times per week for five weeks. Prescription three was used one to two times per week for an additional four weeks. Ear acupuncture was added to help him quit smoking, using Ear Shenmen, Lung 1 and Lung 2, Diaphragm, Subcortex, Stomach, Large Intestine, and Sympathetic nerve.

Herbs
Ping Wei San (Calm the Stomach Powder) and Wei-tai "999" capsules[1] were given.

Results
After the first week of treatment, the patient's headache and stomach symptoms were reduced by 60%. At that time, he attended a party where he drank alcohol and overate. This caused his symptoms to return. Another two weeks of treatment was required to re-stabilize his condition. After and additional four weeks of treatment, his stomach pain and headache were completely gone. He was concurrently treated with ear acupuncture to help him quit smoking. The patient was advised to strictly avoid the foods and drinks which caused his symptoms.

---
[1] A patent formula for gastritis, peptic ulcer, and duodenal ulcer.

Analysis

This case shows the successful application of Stomach, Spleen, Yin Wei and Chong Channel theory. The patient's Yang Ming headache was related to the stomach disorder. The stomach pain was due to accumulation of Damp Heat, and Qi and Blood stagnation in the Middle Jiao, which further resulted in rebellion of Stomach Qi. This blocked the ascension of clear Qi, allowing the turbid Qi to rise, and resulting in the Yang Ming headache.

In the first prescription, the combination of St 30, a Sea of Nutrition point, and St 37, a Sea of Blood point and Lower He (Sea) point of Large Intestine, strongly reverses the rebellion of Stomach Qi. It also promotes normal digestion. LI 11 and Sp 6 clear Damp Heat and nourish the Stomach and Spleen. Ren 10 is a local point for removing obstruction of Stomach Qi, and directing it downward. Yintang is a local point for Yang Ming headache.

In the second prescription, the combination of Sp 4 and Sp 5 with Pc 5 and Pc 6, strongly harmonizes the Stomach and Spleen and regulates the Yin Wei and Chong Channels. St 43, the Shu (Stream) point, regulates the Stomach Qi and stops Yang Ming headache. St 8 is a local point for Yang Ming headache.

In the third prescription, the combination of Ren 12, UB 20, and UB 21 (Front Mu and Back Shu points), harmonize the Middle Jiao, and strengthens the Stomach. UB 17, the Diaphragm Shu point and Influential Point of Blood, opens the Qi in the Middle Jiao and harmonizes rebellion of Qi. GB 30 powerfully opens all the channels, and harmonizes Wood and Earth. St 36 strengthens the Middle Jiao, and helps reduce the patient's sensitivity to foods.

Case 16   Enuresis

Case History

An eight year old boy had wet the bed for several years. His enuresis was more likely to occur if he became over-excited or exhausted during the daytime. His hair looked thin and without normal luster. He had difficulty concentrating in school. Other symptoms included frequent attacks of allergic asthma in the Winter and Spring, poor appetite, occasional poor sleep, and sallow complexion. When he ate dairy products, his symptoms became worse.

Examination

Tongue:	Small, slightly pale and purple, with a sticky coating in the center.
Pulse:	Thready and weak at the Chi regions, wiry at the right Cun region.
Palpation:	Softness and a feeling of emptiness at Ren 4 and UB 23.

Diagnosis

TCM:	Deficiency of Qi of the Kidney, Lung, and Spleen, accumulation of dampness in the Middle Jiao.
WM:	Enuresis.

Principle of Treatment

1) Tonify Qi of the Kidney and Lung, strengthen the Spleen.
2) Resolve Dampness.

Prescription
Acupuncture
1) ᴸ Lu 7 ^Q   ᴿ Ki 6 ^{T & Q}   Ren 4 ^X   Du 4 ^X

2) ᴮ St 36 ^T   ᴮ UB 23 ^{T X & Q}   Du 3 ^{T & X}   ᴮ UB 13 ^{T & Q}

      Tonification with needles for children is performed with ***brushing method*** on each point, 30-50 times. The two groups of points were used in alternation, twice weekly for two months. *Nieji*[1] massage was also performed on the Du Channel and Huatoujiaji line, from the coccyx to C 7.

Results
      After the first week of treatment, the boy did not wet his bed. In the third week of treatment, there was a recurrence of symptoms after he drank a lot of fluids late at night. He was advised not to drink fluids for three hours before going to bed. After he began following this advise, there was steady improvement in all his symptoms. Treatments were continued once every two to three weeks for consolidation of his Lung and Kidney Qi. As the patient's treatments were performed during the Summer, there was no immediate demonstration of improvement in his allergic asthma, however, during the following Winter and Spring, he had only two mild colds with cough, which were quickly cured by herbal treatment.

Analysis
      This is an example of combining both Channel Theory and Zang Fu Theory. The patient's enuresis involved the Lung, Ren, and Du Channels, and an underlying congenital Deficiency of Kidney Qi. UB 13, UB 23, Ki 6, and Lu 7, with intradermal needles, tonify and harmonize the Lung and Kidney Qi, the upper and lower source of water. Moxibustion was used on Ren 4, Du 4, and Du 3 to warm up the Kidney Yang, strengthen the Kidney Qi and Essence, and control the urine. St 36 strengthens the Middle Jiao and resolves Dampness.

      Brushing technique is often used for tonification in the treatment of children. Nieji massage is very effective for strengthening the body constitution, promoting the function of the Du, Ren, and Kidney Channels, and is very good for children with chronic deficiency.

Case 17   Schizophrenia (Dian Kuang Syndrome)

Case History
      A man in his forties was diagnosed as schizophrenic, and had been taking strong doses of lithium and sedatives on an off for several years. His symptoms included constant headache, poor sleep, frequent outbursts of anger, a red face with constant sweating, strong body odor, staring, and a dull look in the eyes. He also suffered from stomach pain, dry mouth, constipation, lower back pain, and knee joint soreness. He talked incessantly. Due to his illness, he had been unable to work at his trade as a construction worker.

Examination
Tongue: Red with redder spots, very dry with cracks, thick, yellow, and unsmooth coating.
Pulse: Forceful, rolling, and wiry, sometimes irregular. Slightly weak with deep pressure at the
                 Chi regions.
Palpation: His abdomen was distended, with tenderness at St 25. The muscles along the Yang

---

[1] This refers to a method of massage. Pinching the skin and flesh with the fingers along the spine, and rolling upward.

Channels on the lower extremities and the Du Channel were very tight. The area of the Huatoujiaji points was very spasmed and elevated.

Diagnosis
TCM: Dian Kuang Syndrome due to Phlegm Fire stirring up Stomach Fire, which disturbs the Mind, Disharmony between the Heart and Stomach

WM: Schizophrenia.

Principle of Treatment
1) Clear Phlegm Fire in the Heart, extinguish Fire in the Stomach.
2) Sedate and calm the Mind, harmonize the Heart and Stomach nourish the Yin.

Prescription
Acupuncture
1) ^{L} St 40 $^{\perp}$ ^{R} Pc 5 $^{\perp}$ Ren 15 $^{\perp}$ ^{R} Ht 8 $^{\perp}$ ^{L} St 44 $^{\perp}$ ^{R} Lv 2 $^{\perp}$ Huatuojiaji pts $^{\circ}$

2) ^{R} Lv 2 & 3 $^{\perp}$ ^{L} LI 3 & 4 $^{\perp}$ Du 24 $^{\perp}$ Du 2 $^{\perp}$ ^{B} GB 20 ^{l} ^{B} Sp 6 ^{T} Du Channel pts $^{\circ}$

Herbs
Modifications of the following formulas were used: Niu Huang Qing Xin Wan (Cattle Gall Stone Pill to Clear the Heart Pill), Meng Shi Gun Tan Wan (Lapis Chloriti Pill to Eliminate Phlegm), Long Dan Xie Gan Tang (Gentiana Longdancao Pill to Drain the Liver) and Tian Wang Bu Xin Dan (Emperor of Heaven's Special Pill to Tonify the Heart).

Results
The two groups of points were used in alternation, twice a week for a total of four months. After the first treatment, the patient reported feeling "like a human being", meaning not mentally disturbed. During the first few weeks of treatment, he had an increased number of bowel movements, in which a large amount of phlegm fluid was eliminated. He was advised to gradually reduce his medication. After four weeks, he was able to completely discontinue his medication. As a result, his dry mouth improved markedly. He was also able to sleep and concentrated better, and his headaches stopped. After another three months of treatment, he was able to return to work and maintain a normal mental state. He was advised to come for treatment, once a month for follow-ups.

Analysis
This case demonstrates the successful application of Stomach, Heart, and Du Channel Theory. Phlegm Fire was the initial pathogenic factor that stirred up Yang Ming Fire, which then transferred to the Heart through the Stomach Divergent Channel. This resulted in the flaring up of Heart Fire, which disturbed the Mind.

St 40 is a Luo (Connecting) point and also a Ghost Point. It is very effective for resolving Phlegm and its influence goes directly to the brain. When used in combination with Pc 5, another Ghost Point, it eliminates phlegm and calms the Mind. Ht 8, Lv 2, and St 44 are all Ying (Spring) points which strongly drain and clear Fire. Ren 15, the Luo (Connecting) point, is directly connected with the Du Channel. It sedates and calms the mind.

In the second prescription, Du 24 and Du 2 (an upper and lower combination) open the Du Channel and sedate and calm the mind. The combination of Lv 2 and Lv 3, with LI 3 and LI 4, is collectively known as *Double Four Gates*. When these pairs of points are used contralaterally, they have a powerful effect in breaking through stagnation of Liver Qi and promoting the free flow of Qi throughout the body. In my experience, this combination is very effective for all mental disorders. GB 20 promotes brain function, and prevents Fire from transforming into Wind. Sp 6 tonifies the Yin which has been consumed by long term accumulation of Fire. Cupping method on the Huatuojiaji points and the Du Channel promotes circulation, relaxes spasms, and brings toxins and stagnation to the surface.

Case 18   Interstitial Cystitis (Lin Syndrome)

Case History
A male patient, aged 43, worked as a lifeguard. He suffered from a painful, burning sensation before and during urination, accompanied by a pulling sensation in the scrotum. His urine was turbid and yellowish. He also suffered from abdominal spasms, lower back pain, muscle spasms and pain of the lower limbs, and coldness of the hands and feet. His symptoms were exacerbated by exposure to cold water, stress, and eating acidic food. They were relieved by hot baths. He liked cold food and beer. The patient had been treated by numerous steroidal and non-steroidal anti-inflammatory drugs, with little improvement. His urinalysis and urine culture were normal.

Examination
Tongue: Swollen with teeth marks, pale purple with a slight tremor, white sticky coating, thick at the root.

Pulse: Deep, thready, choppy, and wiry. Weak on the right Guan region and both Chi regions.

Palpation: Muscle tension and spasms along both sides of the rib cage and m. rectus abdominus, tightness of the muscles along the spine from T 7 to L 2.

Diagnosis
TCM: Damp Cold accumulating in the Lower Jiao, stagnation of Qi and Blood in the Liver Channel with underlying Kidney Yang Deficiency.

WM: Interstitial cystitis.

Principle of Treatment
1) Eliminate Dampness, expel Cold, remove stagnation from the Liver Channel, smooth urination.
2) Activate the circulation of Qi and Blood in the Lower Jiao, tonify the Kidney Yang.

Prescription
Acupuncture
1) ^{B} Lv 1 ^{Δ3} Ren 12 ↑ ^{L} SJ 4 $^{T\&Δ3}$ ^{R} Lv 3 $^{I\&X}$ ^{R} Lv 5 ^{I} ^{B} St 36 ^{T}
^{R} Ki 16 ↑ ^{L} Ashi on the costal arch, level of St 20 ^{I}

2)   Du 4 ↑ ^{B} UB 18 ^{T} ^{B} UB 23 $^{T\&X}$ ^{R} GB 34 ^{I} ^{L} Ki 9 ^{I} ^{R} Ki 3 ^{T}

Treatment was applied twice a week initially, then once a week as the patient progressed, for a total of six months. The two groups of points were used in alternation. Additional points, such as St 36, Sp 3 and Sp 4, Pc 6, and LI 10, were used as modifications. In the first prescription, Ki 16 and the Ashi point on the costal arch were treated contralaterally. The sides were switched after each few treatments. The Ashi point was treated with oblique, shallow insertion, and vibrating method.

Results
Moxibustion was applied to Lv 1 and Du 4 at the beginning of each treatment, after which the patient always felt an immediate release of his muscle spasms. After two weeks of treatment, the painful urination and abdominal spasms were greatly improved. Despite being warned to avoid acidic foods, he felt so much better that he ate some tomatoes and apples, causing a flare up of his pain. The same treatment was again applied consistently, which after four months, led to the complete relief of his symptoms. The patient continued with maintenance treatments for an two additional months. When he was seen one year later for treatment of an unrelated illness, his symptoms had not returned.

Analysis

This case is an example of the application of the theory of the Du, Liver, Kidney, and Yin Wei Channels. Even when urinalysis does not demonstrate a bacterial infection, abnormal urination with discomfort in this type of patient is still considered a Lin Syndrome in Traditional Chinese Medicine. His condition was due to Damp Cold accumulated in the Lower Jiao, and stagnation in the Liver Channel. Du 4 and Lv 1 were treated with moxibustion to warm the Du and Liver Channels, and to promote circulation in the Lower Jiao and the genital area. The combination of Ren 12, SJ 4, and Lv 3 has an energetic influence on, and conducts Qi circulation to, the Lower Jiao. In my experience, this combination, treated by needles and moxibustion, can be effectively used for interstitial cystitis, endometriosis, ovarian cysts, and fibroid tumors. Lv 5 is the Luo (Connecting) point, which has a direct connection with the genital area. Ki 16 is used in combination with the Ashi point on the costal arch, to break up stagnation and relieve abdominal spasms. St 36 strengthens the Middle Jiao, and resolves Damp Cold.

UB 18 and UB 23, the Back Shu points of the Liver and Kidney, were used in combination with Du 4 and Ki 3 to tonify the Liver and Kidney, warm up and promote the circulation, and remove stagnation. GB 3, when used with Ki 9, the Xi (Cleft) of the Yin Wei Channel, loosens the muscles and expels pathogenic factors at the deepest level.

Case 19   Menopause

Case History

A forty-nine year old female patient had suffered from irregular menstruation for two years. Her menstruation occurred only once every several months. When her menstruation came, the flow was very heavy. Initially, the color would be bright red with large clots, then either turn to light red near the end, or she would spot for many days. She often felt fatigue and dizziness. Her symptoms included abdominal cramps, lower back pain, vaginal dryness, hot flashes which were felt in the chest and face, accompanied by a sensation of heat rushing upward, then followed by palpitations and shortness of breath. She also had night sweats, restlessness, nausea, cold feet, and extreme mood swings occasionally. Her complexion was pale. During the previous year, she had undergone a D. & C. procedure twice to correct the heavy bleeding, but these had been unsuccessful. She had been taking hormone replacement therapy, which did not improve her condition, but did cause weight gain, edema, and breast lumps.

Examination

Tongue: Pale, purplish, dusty color, red and swollen on the sides. A white sticky coating from the center toward the root.

Pulse: Thready and wiry, excessive on left Cun and right Guan regions, both Chi regions were weak.

Palpation: Empty feeling and coldness in the Ren 4 area, exquisite tenderness in the UB 23 and 52 areas, tenderness at UB 9, Ki 6, Sp 6, Lv 8, and Lv 9.

Diagnosis

TCM: Disharmony between Water and Fire, due to deficiency of the Kidney and Liver, deficiency of Liver and Spleen Blood, with Liver Yang Hyperactive.

WM: Menopause.

Principle of Treatment

1) Harmonize Fire and Water, nourish the Kidney and Liver.
2) Tonify the Blood, nourish the Liver and Spleen, pacify Liver Yang.

162

Prescription

Acupuncture

1) ^{L} Ki 6 $^{T\ \&\ \triangle5}$ ^{L} Ki 7 ^{T} ^{L} Ht 3$^\perp$ ^{L} Pc 6 ^{I} ^{R} SJ 5 ^{I} ^{R} GB 39 ^{T}

2) ^{B} UB 11 $^{I\ \&\ \triangle5}$ ^{R} St 37 ^{I} ^{R} St 39 ^{I} ^{L} Sp 4 ^{T} ^{R} Pc 6 ^{I} Ren 17 ^{I}

3) ^{B} UB 20 ^{T} ^{B} UB 18 ^{T} ^{B} UB 23 ^{T} ^{B} UB 9 ^{I} ^{B} Lv 3 ^{I} ^{B} Kidney Essence point $^{\triangle5\ \&\ Q}$

Treatments were performed three times a week for the first two weeks, then once or twice a week for two and a half months. The three prescriptions were used in alternation. Additional points, such as Sp 1, Lv 9, Du 4, and Ren 4, were treated with moxa when the patient was hemorrhaging.

Herbs

Modifications of the following formulas were used: An Chong Tang (Calm Uterine Bleeding Decoction), Er Xian San (Two Immortals Powder), Tian Wang Bu Xin Dan (Emperor of Heaven's Special Pill to Tonify the Heart), and Ba Zhen Wan (Eight Treasure Pill).

Results

The patient had heavy bleeding at the time of her first visit. She was immediately treated by moxibustion on Sp 1 and Du 4, followed by acupuncture on Lv 9 and Ren 4, then An Chong Tang (Calm Uterine Bleeding Decoction) was administered. Her bleeding was greatly reduced afterward. The patient was very happy with the result, which was far better than that of the D. & C. Regular acupuncture treatments began from her second visit. After one month of treatment, all her symptoms gradually improved, and she had a regular menstrual period. At the end of the third month of treatment, all her symptoms disappeared, except for occasional, mild, hot flashes, which occurred only after eating. She was advised to take maintenance treatments once every few weeks, do self massage, and to take Er Xian San once a day.

Analysis

This case mainly applies the theory of the Kidney, Chong, Ren, Liver, and Spleen Channels. The patient was in her menopausal transition period, with a variety of complaints. Although her symptoms involved many organs and channels, the declining of Kidney Essence and Qi, and the emptiness of the Chong and Ren Channels, were the main cause. Treating *Ben*, i.e, tonifying the Kidney, Spleen, and Liver, was the key principle of treatment for this case.

In the first prescription, Ki 6 and Ki 7 tonify and strengthen the Kidney, and nourish Water. When used in combination with Ht 3 and Pc 6 they eliminate Heart Fire and harmonize Water and Fire. GB 39, in combination with SJ 5, strengthens the Kidney Essence, promotes the bone marrow, smoothes the flow of Qi in the Three Jiaos, and pacifies Liver Yang.

The second prescription regulated menstruation. UB 11, St 37, and St 39 are the Sea of Blood points. Together with Sp 4 and Pc 6, they regulate the Chong and Ren Channels, and tonify the Liver, Spleen, and Kidney. Ren 17 was used to harmonize the sensation of heat rushing upward to the chest.

In the third prescription, the Back Shu points of the Spleen, Liver, and Kidney, together with the Kidney Essence point, replenish Kidney Essence and Qi, and tonify and strengthen their associated organs. In nearly every patient going through menopause, the Kidney Essence point is exquisitely tender, and should be treated with moxa cones and intradermal needles. UB 9 is at the very end of the Chong Channel, and has a direct relationship with the uterus and adnexa. There is often a strain or tender spot on this point in gynecological disorders. Lv 3 tonifies Liver Blood, pacifies Liver Yang, and soothes Liver Qi to treat mood swings. When there is heavy bleeding, treating *Biao* is the first priority. For this purpose, moxibustion on Sp 1 and Du 4, and acupuncture on Lv 9 and Ren 4, are very effective.

Case 20   Iritis

Case History

A man in his thirties complained of eye pain, with redness and tiredness. Other symptoms included a sandy feeling in his eyes, especially on the right, photophobia, blurring of vision, dry eyes, and sometimes a distending, ocular pain. He also complained of a headache, which radiated from his eyebrow to the temporal and occipital regions. He often felt discomfort in the epigastrium and abdomen, and had loose stools.

The patient's condition was usually aggravated by overeating, especially by sweet and greasy foods, and he had a sticky taste in his mouth. He lived very close to the ocean, and although his life was not especially difficult he worried constantly and was easily depressed. Two years ago, he had a similar attack in his left eye which was unsuccessfully treated by another acupuncturist, who prescribed Liver tonics.

Examination

Tongue: Swollen, pale, dusty looking, with some red spots on the tip. A sticky, yellowish-white coating.

Pulse: Thready, soft, and rolling. Weak when pressed deeply on the left Guan and Chi regions.

Palpation: Tenderness at UB 2 on the right, and at GB 20, LI 4, and Lv 3 bilaterally, muscle tension along the neck and m. trapezius on the right side.

Diagnosis

TCM: Obstruction of the eyes due to: a) Damp Heat contracted in the Gall Bladder, Liver, Stomach, and Spleen Channels, and b) Qi and Blood stagnation of the Liver and Heart. Deficiency of the Liver, Kidney, and Spleen.

WM: Iritis.

Principle of Treatment

1) Eliminate Damp Heat, remove Qi and Blood stagnation, clear the eyes.
2) Strengthen the Liver, Spleen and Heart, brighten the eyes.

Prescription

Acupuncture

1) ^{R} Sp 2 $^\perp$	^{L} SJ 2 $^\perp$	^{L} SI 6 $^\perp$	^{R} Ht 5 ^{I}	^{R} UB 1 ^{I}	^{B} Sp 9 $^\perp$
2) ^{L} LI 4 $^\perp$	^{L} LI 11 ^{I}	^{R} Lv 3 $^\perp$	^{L} GB 37 ^{I}	^{R} Sp 6 ^{T}	^{B} GB 20 ^{I}
3) ^{B} UB 18 ^{T}	^{B} UB 20 ^{T}	^{B} UB 23 ^{T}	^{B} GB 20 ^{I}	^{B} Ki 6 ^{T}	Du 4 ^{TX}

Treatment was given twice a week for five weeks. The three groups of points were used in alternation. Gentle tapping method with a Seven Star Needles was applied along the edge of the ocular orbit at the beginning of each treatment. One or two local points, such as GB 1, UB 2, UB 7, and Du 23, were added each time.

Herbs

Modifications of the following herbal prescriptions were used: Chai Ping Tang (Minor Bupleurum and Calm the Stomach Powder Decoction), Long Dan Xie Gan Tang (Gentiana Longdancao Decoction to Drain the Liver), and Liu Jun Zi Tang plus Ming Mu Di Huang Wan (Six Gentlemen Decoction plus Rehmannia Six Brighten the Eyes Pill).

Results

After one week of treatment, his eye pain was greatly reduced. At the end of the second week, his blurred vision, the sandy feeling in his eyes, and his stomach discomfort was gone. He was advised to strictly avoid sweet and greasy foods, and emotionally stressful situations. At the end of the fifth week, he was completely cured.

Analysis

This case demonstrates the importance of correct differentiation according to channel pathology. This was the second time the patient had had an episode of iritis. He had been given Liver tonics, such as Ji Ju Di Huang Wan (Rehmannia Six with Chrysanthemum and Fructus Lycii), Ming Mu Di Huang Wan (Rehmannia Six Brighten the Eyes Pill), and Shi Hu Ye Gung Wan (Dendrobia Pill for Night Vision) for the first attack. These had little effect, and his recover had been slow.

It should be noted that the Liver is not the only channel which affects the condition of the eye. The eye is connected to all Five Zang organs and their regular channels, plus the Ren, Du, Yin Qiao, and Yang Qiao Channels, the Heart Divergent Channel, and the Heart Luo Collateral. In this case, the patient's eye disorder was due to Damp Heat, transmitted to the eyes related to the Liver, Gall Bladder, Stomach, and Spleen Channels.

In prescription one, the combination of Sp 2 and SJ 2, the Ying (Spring) points, clears Heat and lubricates the eyes. SI 6 and Ht 5 brighten the eyes. Sp 9 resolves dampness and strengthens the Middle Jiao. UB 1was used as a local point.

In the second prescription, LI 4 and LI 11 clear Damp Heat and benefit the eyes. Lv 3 and GB 37 are a Yuan (Source) and Luo (Connecting) combination for soothing the Liver, and nourishing the eyes. Sp 6 nourishes the Kidney and Liver Yin. GB 20 was used as a local point to promote circulation in the eyes.

In the third prescription, the Back Shu points of the Liver, Spleen, and Kidney were treated in combination with Du 4 and Ki 6, to nourish the Liver, tonify the Kidney, strengthen the Spleen, and restore the function of the eyes. Another name for Du 4 is *Jing Ming,* which means "Brighten the Eyes". Tonifying this point with moxibustion directly nourishes the eyes when there are no obvious heat signs.

Glossary

Ben and Biao
These are the terms used for diagnosis and differentiation. They are understood in relationship to each other. For example, Ben means the root cause of the disorder, a deeper penetration of pathogenic factor, and chronic conditions. Biao means the symptoms and signs of the disease, pathogenic factors in the superficial layers, and acute disease.

Bi Jue
Bi means the arm. In general, Jue means cold hands and feet. In the channel pathology of the Nei Jing, Jue means an abnormal condition. Bi Jue, as a syndrome, refers to a group of symptoms and signs which indicate the disorders of the Lung Channel.

Brushing method
This refers to a technique of gently brushing the skin with a single needle. It is often used in the treatment of children.

Dian Kuang
Dian Kuang is a syndrome which expresses itself as violent, out of control behavior.

Double Four Gates
This refers to the combination of Lv 2 and Lv 3 with LI 3 and LI 4.
When these pairs of points are used contralaterally they have a powerful effect in breaking through stagnation of Liver Qi, promoting the free flow of Qi throughout the body.

Eye system
The Eye system includes the tissues, nerves and vessels around and behind the eyes which directly relate to the brain.

Five Wheel Theory
A system of diagnosis observation of the eyes. The pupil corresponds to the Kidney (Water Wheel), the iris to the Liver (Wind Wheel), the sclera to the Lung (Qi Wheel), the Spleen to the upper and lower eyelids (Flesh Wheel), the inner and outer canthi to the Heart (Blood Wheel).

Gan Jue
Gan means the shin area. In general, Jue means cold hands and feet. In the channel pathology of the Nei Jing, Jue means an abnormal condition. Gan Jue, as a syndrome, refers to a group of symptoms and signs which indicate the disorders of the Stomach Channel.

Ghost points
There are thirteen Ghost Points which are used for mental disorders. Sun Si Miao, in the book *Qian Jin Yao Fang*, lists Du 26, Lu 11, Sp 1, Pc 7, UB 62, Du 16, St 6, Ren 24, Pc 8, Du 23, Ren 1, LI 11, and Jin Jin/Yu Ye (extra points). A later generation added two points: Pc 5 and SI 3.

Gu Jue
Gu means the bones. In general, Jue means cold hands and feet. In the channel pathology of the Nei Jing, Jue means an abnormal condition. Gu Jue, as a syndrome, refers to a group of symptoms and signs which indicate the disorders of the bones and the Gall Bladder Channel.

Heart system
The Heart system includes the pericardium, arteries, nerves and tissues surrounding the heart.

Huai Jue
Huai means the ankle. In general, Jue means cold hands and feet. In the channel pathology of the Nei Jing, Jue means an abnormal condition. Huai Jue, as a syndrome, refers to a group of symptoms and signs which indicate the disorders of the Urinary Bladder Channel.

Jie
The distribution of the Tendinomuscular Channels can be summarized in four words: Jie (knot), Ju (convergences), Luo (connect) - San (dispersion). The Qi and blood of each Tendinomuscular Channel concentrates at certain areas, generally at large muscles or joints. The *Jie* concentrations are especially important and will be designated by the term knot when the pathways of each individual Tendinomuscular Channels are described.

Jin Ye	These two terms refer to the Body fluids. The Jin is called "thin", like urine, sweat, tears, and saliva. The Ye is more turbid like lubricating fluids, e.g. synovial.
Jing Luo Longyanxue	Jing Lou means swelling and pain of the lymph glands along the sides of the neck. Longyanxue means "Point of the Eye of the Dragon". It is located on the Small Intestine Channel on the small finger. Flex the finger, then take the point at the end of the skin crease on the lateral aspect at the junction of the first and second proximal phalanges.
Nieji massage	This refers to a method of massage. Pinching the skin and flesh with the fingers along the spine, and rolling upward.
Pertaining and Connecting	There are six pairs of Yin and Yang Channels which form a specific relationship, externally and internally. The Yin Channels are said to "pertain" to the Zang organs, and be "connected" to the Fu organs of their Yang paired channels. The Yang Channels are said to "pertain" to the Fu organs, and be "connected" to the Zang organs of their Yin paired channels.
Pi Zheng	This refers distention and fullness sensation in the epigastrium due to non-substantial accumulation. It is a stagnation of Qi which is not painful with pressure. It is typically treated with Ban Xia Xie Xin Tang (Pinellia Decoction to Drain the Epigastrium).
Qi Jie	Jie means "Street". There are two meanings for Qi Jie. The first is the broad concept of where Qi accumulates in the body. There are four main areas head, chest, abdomen (including the back) and the shin. The other meaning refers to the area of the inguinal groove, approximately St 30 (Qichong).
Shan	Shan means hernia. There are seven types of hernia mentioned in the Nei Jing, but little explanation is offered. Later generations detailed the description of these disorders. The material in this text is from those sources, i.e., Zhu Bing Yuan Hou Lun (Treatise on the Sources and Explanation of all Diseases), I Zhong Bi Du (Essential Medical Book).
Sky Window	This refers to the points that have the word "Tian" (which means heaven) in their name. They are often used to treat the disorders of the head and face, and are also effective for releasing mental and emotional stress. There are sixteen points altogether: Lu 3, LI 17, St 25, Sp 18, SI 11, SI 16, SI 17, UB 7, UB 10, Pc 1, Pc 2, SJ 15, SJ 16, SJ 10, GB 9, and Ren 22. Some texts also list St 9 as a Sky Window point.
TDP lamp	Physiotherapeutic device which produces a combination of heat and magnetic waves, which can penetrate into the deeper layers of the tissues.
Yang Jue	Yang refers the Yang Qi. In general, Jue means cold hands and feet. In the channel pathology of the Nei Jing, Jue means an abnormal condition. Yang Jue, as a syndrome, refers to a group of symptoms and signs which indicate the disorders of the Gall Bladder Channel.
Zhen Jia	Zhen means substantial accumulation and growth, such as tumors, carcinomas, cysts, nodules, and fibroids. Jia means accumulations which are primarily due to Qi stagnation, such as Qi masses.
Zheng Zhong	Zheng Zhong refers to an extreme case of palpitation as if a person were frightened or startled.

Bibliography

1982 The Yellow Emperor's Classic of Internal Medicine-Simple Questions (Huang Di Nei Jing Su Wen Jiao Shi). People's Health Publishing House, Beijing, PRC.

1981 Spiritual Axis (Huang Di Nei Jing Ling Shu Jing). People's Health Publishing House, Beijing, PRC

1979 A Revised Explanation of the Classic of difficulties Nanjing College of Traditional. (Nan Jing Jiao Shi). Nanjing College of traditional Chinese Medicine. People's Health Publishing House, Beijing, PRC.

1980 Compendium of Acupuncture (Zhen Jiu Da Cheng). Yang Ji Zhou. People's Health Publishing House, Beijing, PRC.

1982 Essential Collection of Acupuncture Points from the ABC of Acupuncture (Zhen Jiu Jia Yi Jing Shu Xue Zhong Ji). Zhang Shan Chen. Shandong Scientific Publishing House, Shandong, PRC.

1987 Chinese Acupuncture and Moxibustion. Chief editor Chen Xinnong. Foreign Languages Press, Beijing, PRC.

1981 Acupuncture: A Comprehensive Text. John O'Connor and Dan Bensky. Eastland Press, Chicago, Ill.

Additional material taken from the lectures of Yitian Ni, 1978 - 1994.

Index

178